Edited by E.I. Hernández-Jiménez

BOTULINUM TOXIN

IN COSMETIC DERMATOLOGY & SKINCARE PRACTICE

Cosmetics & Medicine
Publishing

Author/Editor:

Elena I. Hernández-Jiménez, *Ph.D.*

Contributors:

Yana A. Yutskovskaya, *M.D., Ph.D., Prof*. Dermatologist

Alisa A. Sharova, *M.D., Ph.D., Associate professor*. Dermatologist, gerontologist

Alena N. Saromytskaya, *M.D.* Dermatologist, laser therapist

BOTULINUM TOXIN IN COSMETIC DERMATOLOGY AND SKINCARE PRACTICE

Botulinum therapy occupies a special place in modern aesthetic medicine, not only as one of the most effective methods with more than 30 years of successful medical history but also as a tool that raises many questions. However, all known medical books on botulinum therapy primarily consider practical aspects — determination of injection points, dosage, etc. While this is certainly valuable information for botulinum therapy practitioners, everyone else is more concerned with other issues — whether botulinum toxin is safe, how it works, what effects can be expected from its use, and how to maximize its duration.

These and other essential questions are addressed in our book — no one has ever dealt with botulinum toxin and its possibilities in such detail! We will identify the critical points related to botulinum toxin and its use in clinical practice. After discussing the nature of the active ingredient — botulinum toxin — we will move on to a brief review of commercial preparations, followed by the main factors affecting the treatment efficacy and safety, backed up by references to authoritative scientific studies. We will outline and justify the main directions of applying botulinum toxin for aesthetic and dermatological indications. We will also discuss the specifics of combining botulinum therapy with other injectable and device-based methods within the framework of complex aesthetic programs for the prevention and correction of age-related skin changes.

This book is part of the *Cosmetic Dermatology & Skincare Practice* book series, covering the most relevant topics in modern dermatology and aesthetic medicine. All books are structured, written in accessible language, and answer critical questions about the problem or technology at hand.

The information in this book will be useful to aestheticians, dermatologists, physiotherapists, neurologists, ophthalmologists, and plastic surgeons — both practicing and those just beginning to master botulinum therapy — as well as medical students and all interested parties.

ISBN 978-1-970196-32-0 (paperback)

ISBN 978-1-970196-36-8 (hardcover)

ISBN 978-1-970196-31-3 (eBook — Adobe PDF)

ISBN 978-1-970196-35-1 (eBook — ePUB)

FirstEditing

English version is edited and certified by the FirstEditing.Com, Inc. (USA).

Author/Editor

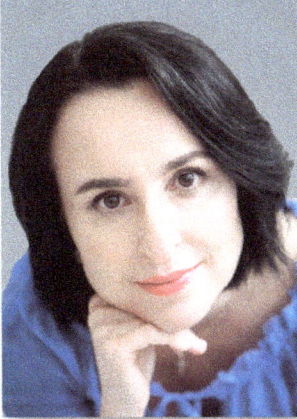

Elena I. Hernández-Jiménez, *Ph.D.*

Biophysicist, scientific journalist

Editor-in-chief of Cosmetics and Medicine Publishing

Chairperson of the Executive Board of the International Society of Applied Corneotherapy (I.A.C.)

Author and co-author of numerous publications in professional magazines, co-author and editor of the book series *Fundamentals of Cosmetic Dermatology & Skincare, Cosmetic Dermatology & Skincare Practice, Cosmetic Chemistry for Dermatology & Skincare Specialists* and others

Speaker at international conferences, author of training seminars and webinars for professionals in the field of skincare

Professional interests: biology and physiology of the skin, skin permeability, cosmetic chemistry, anti-age medicine, physiotherapy in dermatology and aesthetic medicine, skin analysis and imaging

Table of Contents

PART III

BOTULINUM TOXIN AND SKIN HEALTH

PART IV

COMBINING BOTULINUM THERAPY
WITH AESTHETIC TREATMENTS

Abbreviations

α-SMA — smooth muscle alpha-actin
ACh — acetylcholine
AGA — androgenetic alopecia
AMF — age marker fascicles
ASPS — American Society of Plastic Surgeons
ATP — adenosine triphosphate
bFGF — basic fibroblast growth factor
BoNT — botulinum neurotoxin
BoNT/A — botulinum neurotoxin type A
BoNT/B — botulinum neurotoxin type B
CGRP — calcitonin gene-related peptide
CT — computer tomography
DAO — *depressor anguli oris* muscle
DHT — dihydrotestosterone
DOPA — dihydroxyphenylalanine
EMS — electromyostimulation
ERK — extracellular signal-regulated kinase
FDA — U.S. Food and Drug Administration
ICD — International Classification of Diseases
IL — interleukin
INCI — International Nomenclature of Cosmetic Ingredients
IPL — intense pulsed light
KLK-5 — kallikrein-5
LLLT — low-level laser (light) therapy
MMP — matrix metalloproteinase
MRI — magnetic resonance imaging
NO — nitric oxide
PDGFA — platelet-derived growth factor subunit A
PG — prostaglandin
PMF — pulsed magnetic field
PRAR-γ — peroxisome proliferator-activated receptor gamma
PRP — platelet-rich plasma

RF	— radiofrequency
ROS	— reactive oxygen species
RSNA	— Radiological Society of North America
SMAS	— superficial muscular aponeurotic system
SNARE	— soluble N-ethylmaleimide-sensitive factor activating protein receptor
SOD	— superoxide dismutase
SP	— substance P
TGF-β	— transforming growth factor beta
TLR	— toll-like receptor
TNFα	— tumor necrosis factor α
TRP	— transient receptor potential channels
TRPV	— transient receptor potential vanilloid subtype
UV	— ultraviolet
UVA	— ultraviolet type A
UVB	— ultraviolet type B
VEGF	— vascular endothelial growth factor

Introduction

Botulinum therapy occupies a special place in modern aesthetic medicine. This purely therapeutic method, used for severe medical indications, was unexpectedly discovered to exhibit the capacity to solve aesthetic problems better than any traditional cosmetic approach.

However, despite more than 30 years of successful application, physicians and their patients have different attitudes towards this botulinum use. Here, we can find the entire spectrum of emotions and opinions — from complete rejection and fear to enthusiasm, expecting a miracle. Both extremes are related to stereotypes and lack of awareness.

Accordingly, the main objective of our book is to present this truly unique method comprehensively and objectively, helping justify its widespread adoption by cosmetic dermatologists and plastic surgeons.

And not only by them! In fact, botulinum toxin (BoNT) injections were first used in ophthalmology and neurology, and in many cases, they still remain the only alternative.

BoNT refers to substances with a nerve-paralyzing effect. It blocks the signal transmission from the nerve endings to the muscle, preventing the command to contract from reaching the muscle. As a result, it remains relaxed — up to complete paralysis. This effect is reversible, as innervation is restored after some time. As the degree of relaxation of the target muscle can be precisely controlled by the administered dose, BoNT makes it possible to solve a wide range of problems associated with muscle spasms.

Botulinum toxin received the first official recognition as a drug in December 1989 (Scott A.B. et al., 2023): a formulation of Oculinum® (botulinum neurotoxin type A, BoNT/A) was authorized by the U.S. Food and Drug Administration (FDA) for the treatment of strabismus, hemifacial spasm, and blepharospasm in patients older than 12 years of age (**Fig. I-1**).

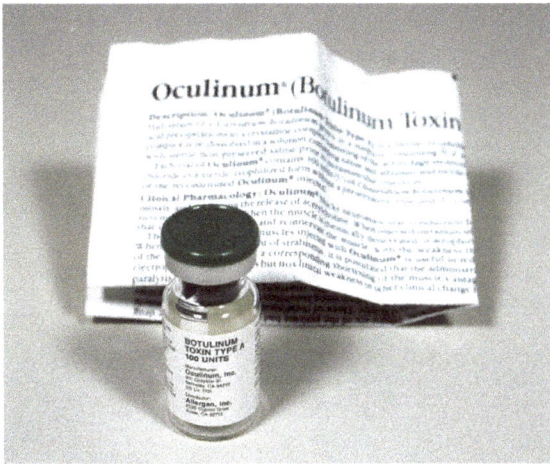

Figure I-1. Oculinum®: the first commercial preparation of botulinum toxin type A

Two years later, in 1991, Allergan, the company that owned the rights to manufacture and distribute the drug, changed its name to Botox. The change was significant — it made it clear that the range of BoNT applications was much broader than ophthalmic problems.

Table I-1 provides a partial list of neurologic indications for BoNT use. These include dystonia in various diseases, muscle spasticity

Table I-1. BoNT applications in medicine

SYMPTOM	DISORDER
Dystonia	Blepharospasm, cervical dystonia, pharyngolaryngeal dystonia, oromandibular dystonia, limbic and axial dystonias, etc.
Spasticity	Cerebral palsy, concussion, post-traumatic spasticity, multiple sclerosis, spinal cord injury
Hemifacial spasm	Facial nerve compression
Overactive sweat glands	Local hyperhidrosis, profuse salivation, Frey syndrome, crocodile tears syndrome, tremor, myokymia
Pain syndrome	Fibromyalgia, pear muscle syndrome (piriformis syndrome), radiculopathy, spinal muscle spasm
Bladder dysfunction	Detrusor sphincter dyssynergia, detrusor hyperreflexia
Eyeball movement disorders	Nystagmus, chronic paralysis of the VI nerve
Others	Stuttering, facial nerve damage, bruxism (teeth grinding during sleep), stilted gait

2002	2004
FDA approval obtained for the use of botulinum toxin type A for the correction of glabellar wrinkles (Image by Freepik)	FDA approval for botulinum toxin type A for the treatment of axillary hyperhidrosis (adapted from Lakraj A.A.D. et al., 2013)

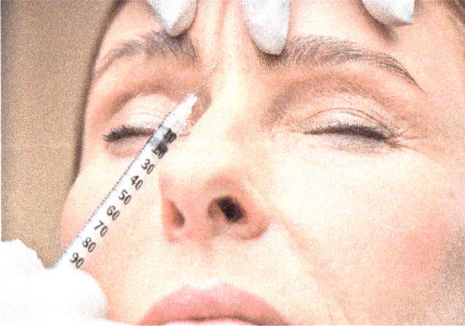

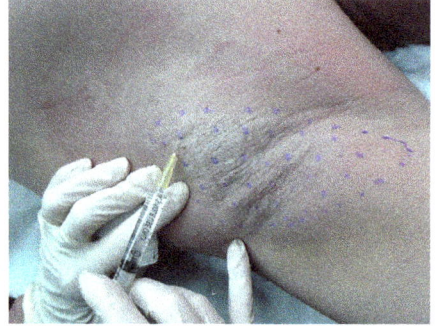

Figure I-2. Official opening of the era of botulinum therapy in aesthetic medicine

(including in cerebral palsy and multiple sclerosis), hemifacial spasms in facial nerve compression, pain syndrome, bladder dysfunction, and many others.

Currently, botulinum therapy is widely used for 150 different indications, often beyond the official guidelines. Their inclusion in the official list is a matter of time, which is necessary to gather the evidence base.

At the same time, several aesthetic indications are already on this list. In 2002, the FDA approved BoNT injection to correct glabellar wrinkles; in 2004, it was approved for treating primary axillary hyperhidrosis (**Fig. I-2**). Moreover, in hyperhidrosis, the effect is related to the blockade of signal transmission from the nerve ending to the sweat gland cells rather than to the muscle.

As BoNT is a poison, its production, storage, transportation, and use are strictly controlled. Fewer than 10 companies are currently authorized to manufacture BoNT products worldwide, and there are a limited number of products on the market, some of which are sold under different trade names depending on the market and/or intended applications. Here are some examples:

- **Botox® / Botox Cosmetic® / Visrabel® / Vistabex®**
  Generic name: onabotulinumtoxinA
  Company: Allergan, Inc. (USA)
- **Dysport® / Reloxin® / Azzalura®**
  Generic name: abobotulinumtoxinA
  Company: Ipsen Biopharmaceuticals, Inc. (France)
- **Daxxify® / Daxi®**
  Generic name: daxibotulinumtoxinumtoxinA-lanm
  Company: Revance Therapeutics, Inc. (USA)
- **Jeuveau™**
  Generic name: prabotulinumtoxinA-xvfs
  Company: Evolus, Inc. (USA)
- **Prosigne® / Lantox®**
  Generic name: CBTX-A
  Company: Lanzhou Institute of Biological Products (China)
- **Neuronox®**
  Generic name: BONTA
  Company: Medy-Tox, Inc. (South Korea)
- **MyoBloc® / NeuroBloc®**
  Generic name: rimabotulinumtoxinB
  Company: Solstice Neurosciences Inc. (USA)

In Part I, we will discuss the differences between commercial BoNT products and the main factors determining the effectiveness of botulinum therapy.

Part I

Botulinum toxin — there's only one! The basics of botulinum therapy

This part covers the key points and concepts related to botulinum toxin and its use in clinical practice. We will commence with the nature of the active ingredient — botulinum toxin — and then provide a brief overview of commercial preparations. After that, we will discuss the main factors affecting the treatment efficacy and safety. We will also outline the main areas of application of botulinum toxin for aesthetic indications. This is the basic knowledge necessary to understand the essence of botulinum therapy and its therapeutic possibilities in general (Jabbari B., 2018). Building on this theoretical foundation, one can move on to the practical details — dose calculations, determination of injection points, injection techniques, etc. These critical details and nuances are the kind of professional information that physicians share in publications in the medical press and at professional events that teachers and instructors provide in training courses.

Chapter 1
The nature of botulinum toxin

1.1. Structure of botulinum toxin

BoNT is a protein complex (**Fig. I-1-1**) secreted by the anaerobic Gram-positive spore-forming microorganism *Clostridium botulinum*. The active core of BoNT (the **neurotoxin itself**) consists of two polypeptide chains connected by a disulfide bond.

The composition of the short chain (light, with a molecular mass of about 50 kDa) varies (Dolly J., Aoki K., 2006). Currently, seven serotypes of BoNT and more than 20 subtypes are known. The most potent is type A (BoNT/A) used in aesthetic medicine (Peck M.W. et al., 2017).

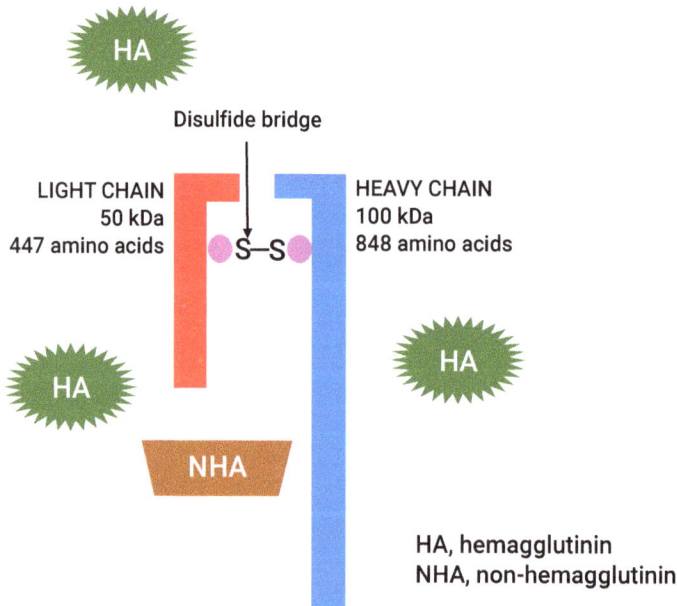

HA

Disulfide bridge

LIGHT CHAIN
50 kDa
447 amino acids

S—S

HEAVY CHAIN
100 kDa
848 amino acids

HA

HA

NHA

HA, hemagglutinin
NHA, non-hemagglutinin

Figure I-1-1. BoNT is composed of light and heavy protein chains surrounded by complexing (stabilizing) proteins

The long chain is also known as the heavy chain, as its molecular mass is twice that of the light chain. The long chain is the same in all BoNT types.

Botulinum toxin complex contains an active neurotoxin and complexing proteins, the latter of which, it is believed, protect the neurotoxin when in the gastrointestinal tract and may facilitate its absorption. Several complex proteins belong to the hemagglutinin group, and one does not.

This entire protein complex is inactive by itself. Removing the defense proteins is not enough to activate it. The active ingredient is the light chain, which must be inside the nerve ending to realize its activity (Choudhury S. et al., 2021).

This phenomenon is discussed next.

1.2. Mechanism of chemical denervation

1.2.1. BoNT penetration and activation in the nerve cell

The complexing proteins detach from the protein complex in the muscle tissue, and the core neurotoxin continues its movement without them (**Fig. I-1-2**).

Once it is near the nerve ending, its heavy chain binds to the appropriate receptor on the cell membrane (**step 1**). At this point, the membrane

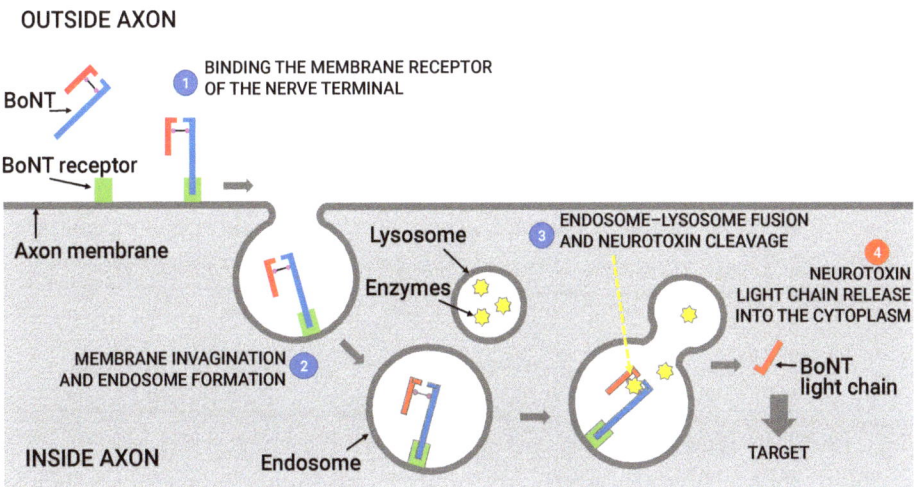

OUTSIDE AXON

BoNT

BoNT receptor

BINDING THE MEMBRANE RECEPTOR
1 OF THE NERVE TERMINAL

Axon membrane

Lysosome

ENDOSOME–LYSOSOME FUSION
3 AND NEUROTOXIN CLEAVAGE

Enzymes

4

NEUROTOXIN
LIGHT CHAIN RELEASE
INTO THE CYTOPLASM

MEMBRANE INVAGINATION
AND ENDOSOME FORMATION 2

←BoNT
light chain

INSIDE AXON

Endosome

TARGET

Figure I-1-2. BoNT penetration and activation inside the axon

segment begins to deepen (invagination) until the edges close over it, and the newly formed vesicle (endosome) with the neurotoxin inside is in the cytoplasm of the nerve cell (**step 2**).

The endosome then fuses with another vesicle, the lysosome, which contains special enzymes (**step 3**). The enzymes cut the disulfide bridge between the heavy and the light chain, and the light chain is set free (**step 4**).

Once in the nerve cell's cytoplasm, the light chain rushes to its target. This target is in the nerve ending, where neurotransmitters (signaling molecules) are released toward the muscle.

So, what is the target, and what happens when it interacts with the light chain of a neurotoxin?

Let's look at the diagram in **Fig. I-1-3** to understand this process.

1.2.2. Blockade of signal transmission from nerve ending to muscle

As shown in **Fig. I-1-3A**, a command is transmitted from a nerve cell to a muscle at a synapse. On the nerve cell side, the synapse is bounded by the presynaptic membrane; on the muscle side, it is bounded by the postsynaptic membrane. The space between the two is called the synaptic cleft.

There is only one command from the nerve ending to the cell — to contract! In the absence of a command, no contraction occurs. This command is transmitted by a substance called a nerve mediator. In this case, it's acetylcholine (ACh).

ACh is produced in the nerve cell and accumulates in special containers — synaptic vesicles. If necessary, the synaptic vesicle approaches the synapse, docks with the presynaptic membrane from the inside, and fuses. As a result, ACh moves outside and ends up in the synaptic cleft. The muscle on the opposite side contains special receptors on its membrane with which ACh binds and triggers the contraction process.

The ACh release is uncontrolled in some conditions and pathologies, such as nerve damage. The muscle is "bombarded" with a flood of signals, and it is in a state of partial (hypertonus) or complete contraction (spasm).

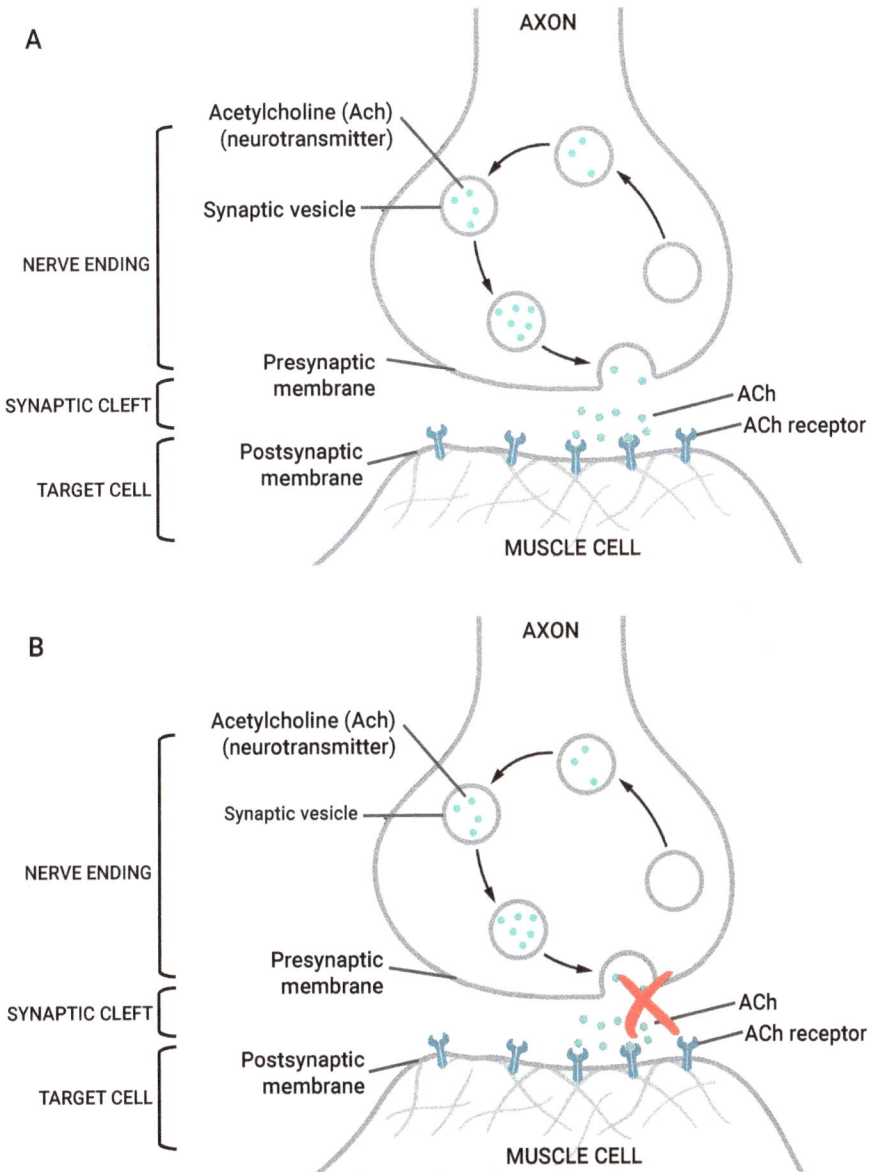

A

AXON

Acetylcholine (Ach)
(neurotransmitter)

Synaptic vesicle

NERVE ENDING

Presynaptic
membrane

SYNAPTIC CLEFT

Postsynaptic
membrane

TARGET CELL

ACh

ACh receptor

MUSCLE CELL

B

AXON

Acetylcholine (Ach)
(neurotransmitter)

Synaptic vesicle

NERVE ENDING

Presynaptic
membrane

SYNAPTIC CLEFT

Postsynaptic
membrane

TARGET CELL

ACh

ACh receptor

MUSCLE CELL

Author: Thomas Splettstoesser (www.scistyle.com)
(figure adapted)

Figure I-1-3. (A) Neuromuscular junction and (B) BoNT site of action

As BoNT blocks the ACh release, the muscle does not receive a signal to contract (**Fig. I-1-3B**).

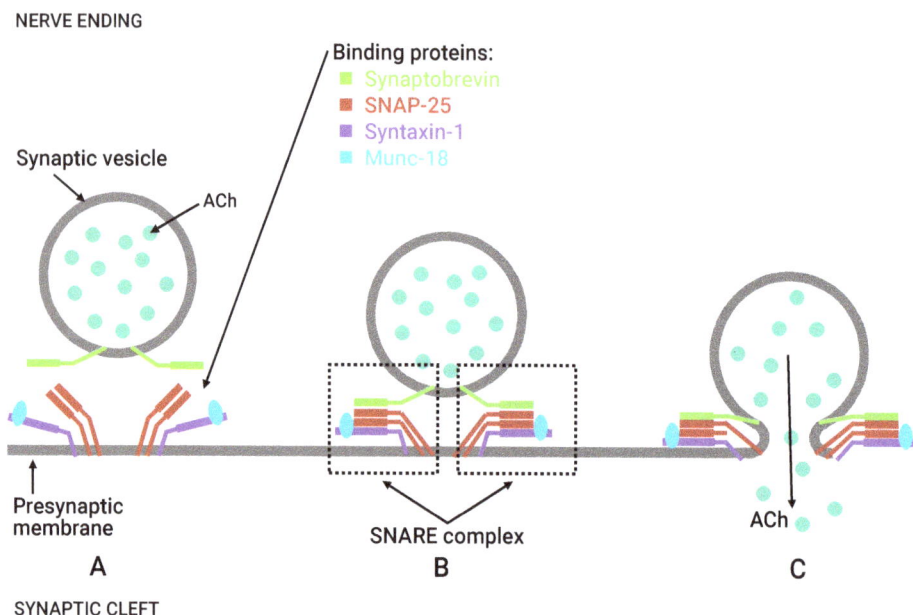

NERVE ENDING

Binding proteins:
- Synaptobrevin
- SNAP-25
- Syntaxin-1
- Munc-18

Synaptic vesicle

ACh

Presynaptic
membrane

SNARE complex

ACh

A   B   C

SYNAPTIC CLEFT

Figure I-1-4. Signal transmission from a nerve ending to a target

This process is depicted in **Fig. I-1-4**. The synaptic vesicle must first bind to the presynaptic membrane for mediator release. Special proteins — some of which are located on the vesicle membrane and others on the presynaptic membrane — assist the binding (**Fig. I-1-4A**). When the synaptic vesicle is sufficiently far from the presynaptic membrane, the proteins dock to form a unique protein complex, the so-called SNARE-complex* (**Fig. I-1-4B**). It ensures close contact between the vesicle and the membrane with the subsequent formation of a channel through which ACh will exit outward into the synaptic cleft (**Fig. I-1-4C**).

The BoNT light chain is a zinc-dependent protease that selectively degrades one of the SNARE proteins (**Fig. I-1-5**). For BoNT/A, this is SNAP-25; for other types of BoNT, it will be other proteins. However, the result of this disruption will be the same: the inability to

———————

*SNARE (soluble N-ethylmaleimide-sensitive factor activating protein receptor) proteins have critical roles in neurotransmitter release and many other forms of membrane fusion. They have been at the forefront of research on biological membrane fusion for some time.

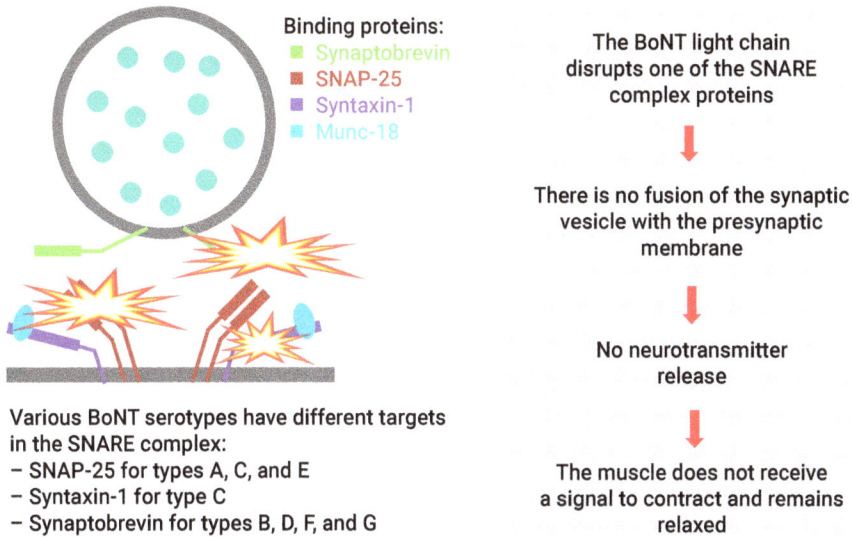

Binding proteins:
- Synaptobrevin
- SNAP-25
- Syntaxin-1
- Munc-18

The BoNT light chain disrupts one of the SNARE complex proteins

↓

There is no fusion of the synaptic vesicle with the presynaptic membrane

↓

No neurotransmitter release

↓

The muscle does not receive a signal to contract and remains relaxed

Various BoNT serotypes have different targets in the SNARE complex:
- SNAP-25 for types A, C, and E
- Syntaxin-1 for type C
- Synaptobrevin for types B, D, F, and G

Figure I-1-5. How botulinum toxin blocks signal transduction

form the latch complex, which means that the synaptic vesicle cannot bind to the membrane, and ACh release and signal transduction are blocked. Since ACh is no longer released, no nerve impulse is delivered to the muscle fiber, and it stops contracting, i.e., it relaxes. This is the general scheme of BoNT action, commonly known as **chemical denervation**.

Chemical denervation of sweat glands occurs similarly. ACh stimulates sweat cell secretory activity. Due to denervation, there is no signal for synthesis, and no sweat is produced.

The process of BoNT introduction into the nerve ending and disruption of synaptic vesicle docking with the presynaptic membrane takes 1–3 days, so the clinical effect begins to manifest several days after the injection (Ledda C. et al., 2022): in small muscles of the face, larynx, and hand — in 2–7 days, in large muscles of the neck, limbs, and trunk — in 7–14 days, and in exocrine glands — in 1–5 days. There are known cases of rapid-onset and delayed effects for 3–4 weeks (Lebeda F.J. et al., 2010).

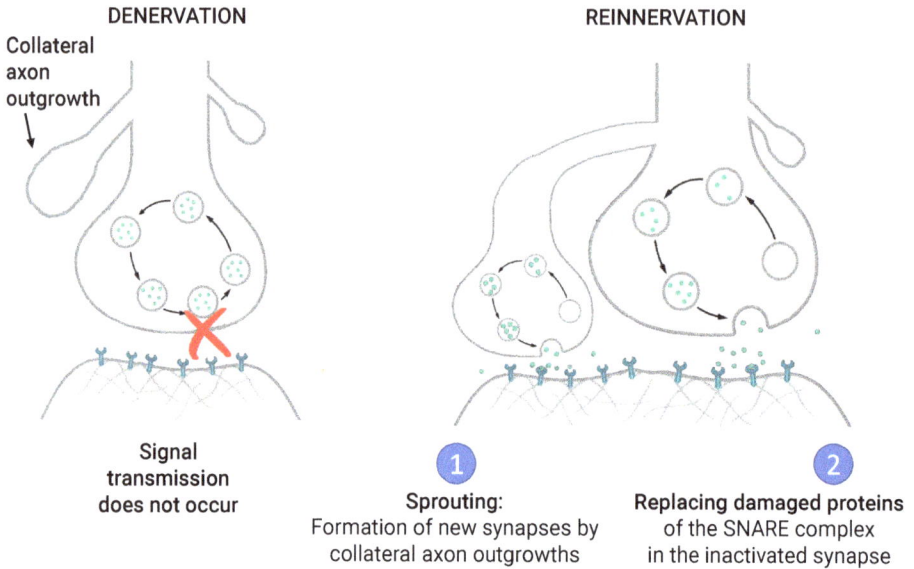

Collateral axon outgrowth

Signal transmission does not occur

1
Sprouting:
Formation of new synapses by collateral axon outgrowths

2
Replacing damaged proteins of the SNARE complex in the inactivated synapse

Figure I-1-6. Denervation and reinnervation processes

1.3. Restoration of innervation

Innervation will be restored after some time, i.e., the clinical effect of the neurotoxin is **reversible** (**Fig. I-1-6**).

BoNT does not affect the anatomical integrity of motor nerve axon terminals, but its administration leads to the same changes as nerve crossing: rapid growth of compensatory terminals is induced — the so-called sprouting (Comella J.X. et al., 1993; Ko C.P., 2008; Rogozhin A.A. et al., 2008). Terminal sprouting is detectable as early as 24 h after BoNT administration. It starts at the sites of myelinated sheath ruptures (so-called Ranvier intercepts) near the inactivated synapse, whereas new terminals are located mainly along the longitudinal axis of denervated muscle fibers.

Simultaneously with the formation of new synapses, the old ones will be restored — the **damaged proteins of the SNARE complex are eventually replaced by new ones**, and the disrupted synapses will start working again. After about 12 weeks, ACh transport through the blocked terminal resumes, and the compensatory innervation terminals will gradually disappear.

Synapse repair requires sufficient amounts of adenosine triphosphate (ATP), specific metabolites, and Ca^{2+} ions (universal messenger in biochemical reactions). Excessive or insufficient Ca^{2+} content is associated with impaired regulation of the fundamental processes of neuron vital activity. Katz and Miledi established the critical role of Ca^{2+} ions in synaptic transmission in the 1960s and proved that Ca^{2+} triggers neurotransmitter release from the presynaptic ending (Katz B., Miledi E., 1967). In recent years, new functions of calcium in synapse physiology have been discovered, including neuronal network formation and the fine regulation of synaptic transmission. Typically, an action potential arriving at the synapse via the presynaptic fiber causes membrane depolarization and activation of the calcium pump. Ca^{2+} ions enter the synapse, bound by the membrane proteins of synaptic vesicles, which promotes active emptying of vesicles into the synaptic cleft. After ACh activation of cholinergic receptors on the postsynaptic membrane of a muscle fiber, protein channels in the membrane open, allowing Na^+ ions to enter the muscle cell. As a result, the muscle cell membrane is depolarized, and the action potential of the muscle fiber is generated.

Chapter 2
Factors that determine the botulinum therapy effectiveness

2.1. Frequently asked questions about the effectiveness of BoNT drugs

2.1.1. Why is BoNT type A used in medicine?

Different toxin serotypes differ in the molecular mechanism of action and the strength of the blocking effect. Owing to its most potent effects, BoNT/A is the most studied. In addition to its myorelaxant effect, BoNT is characterized by an analgesic effect, which is valuable in muscle spasms accompanied by pain.

All commercial preparations registered to date are BoNT type A, except for one — MioBloc® (Solstice Neurosciences, USA; registered in Europe as NeuroBloc®), the active ingredient of which is BoNT type B (BoNT/B). However, MioBloc is not used in aesthetic medicine.

2.1.2. What does the area of denervation depend on?

It depends on the administered BoNT dose.

2.1.3. How long does the effect last after the BoNT administration?

On average, the BoNT injection effects last 3–6 months, but in some cases, they can last longer; for example, this period is extended up to 12 months when treating hyperhidrosis.

2.1.4. Which commercial BoNT product is the most effective?

It is common for patients and physicians to ask about the relative effectiveness of different BoNT drugs on the market.

At first glance, the question seems simple, but the answer is somewhat complicated, as discussed below (Brin M.F. et al., 2024).

First, the preparations differ in the active site (**Table I-2-1**). For example, all preparations except Xeomin contain a botulinum toxin complex that includes hemagglutinin and neurotoxin. Xeomin does not contain hemagglutinin.

Second, each preparation has an additional stabilization system, which may include human albumin, gelatin, dextran, lactose, maltose, and sucrose in various combinations and amounts.

Each manufacturer uses different *Clostridium* strains and technologies for toxin isolation and purification. Purified neurotoxins differ in activity and stability, so the stabilizing system differs in each case.

Differences in composition affect the drug's behavior in the tissue after administration. In this regard, each product has specific recommended therapeutic doses. These doses, expressed in Units of Activity, are product-specific and may differ by several factors. Therefore, the recommended therapeutic dose is not a comparison criterion **but a peculiarity of each product**.

Consequently, rather than pondering on the effectiveness, focus should be given to correct product selection, ensuring that it is a registered product supplied by a legitimate supplier that has been transported and stored correctly and, when using it, the manufacturer's dosage recommendations and the correct administration technique must be strictly followed.

Table 1-2-1. BoNT/A drugs approved for aesthetic injection in the U.S. (Salame N. et al., 2023)

	Daxibot-ulinum-toxinA	Onabotu-linum-toxinA	Abobot-ulinum-toxinA	Incobot-ulinum-toxinA	Prabotu-linum-toxinA
Brand name	Daxi, Daxxify	Botox	Dysport	Xeomin	Jeuveau
Manufac-turer	Revance Therapeu-tics	Allergan Pharma-ceuticals	Ipsen Biopharm	Merz Pharma	Evolus
Packaging (U/vial)	100	100	500	100	100
Constitu-ents and excipients	• RTP004 • Polysor-bate-20 • Sugar • Buffer	• Hema-glutinin and non-hema-glutin proteins • HSA, 500 µg • Saccha-rose • NaCl	• Hema-glutinin and non-hema-glutin proteins • HSA, 125 µg • Lactose	• HSA, 1 mg • Saccha-rose	• HSA • NaCl
Mol. weight (kDa)	150	900	500–900	150	900
Prepara-tion	Lyophiliza-tion	Vacuum-drying	Lyophiliza-tion	Lyophiliza-tion	Vacuum-drying
Storage prior to reconstitu-tion	Room tem-perature	2–8 °C	2–8 °C	Room tem-perature	2–8 °C
Shelf-life once recon-stituted	72 hours	36 hours	24 hours	36 hours	24 hours
Median duration of the clinical effect	6 months	3–4 months	4 months	3 months	1 month

U — units; HSA — human serum albumin; kDa — kilodalton; NaCl — sodium chloride; RTP004 — stabilizing excipient peptide

Besides these technical aspects, due consideration must be given to the **clinical issues** — correct diagnosis and accurate identification of the target muscle. Physicians are taught these essential practical skills as a part of specialized botulinum therapy courses and training programs. Thus, we will not discuss them in this book, but will answer another frequently asked question — why does BoNT injection produce no or insufficient effect in some patients?

2.2. Insensitivity to botulinum toxin

While it is often assumed that any BoNT preparation will achieve the desired effect if the procedure is performed correctly, this is not necessarily true.

It sporadic cases, there is no effect, or it is too weak. This can occur after the first treatment but also following successful long-term botulinum therapy (**Table I-2-2**).

Table I-2-2. The main causes of botulinum therapy's ineffectiveness

PRIMARY INSENSITIVITY	SECONDARY INSENSITIVITY
• Physician error: incorrect diagnosis, target muscle choice, or insertion technique • Low-quality product • Congenital insensitivity	• Psychological factors (depression) • Exacerbation of the underlying disease • Injection technique mistakes and errors • Reduced drug activity • Immunoresistance associated with the formation of neutralizing antibodies

2.2.1. Primary insensitivity

If BoNT did not work the first time, the reason may lie in the drug (purchased from a dubious supplier, expired, violations of the transportation and storage conditions, etc.).

A medical error, such as a misdiagnosis, insufficient dose, or incorrectly determined injection points, can also lead to inadequate effect.

However, some patients may have an inherently reduced sensitivity to BoNT. This is a genetic trait associated, for example, with an altered receptor on the nerve cell membrane to which BoNT binds. The receptor's configuration may be such that it precludes or hinders the BoNT heavy chain binding. If this is the case, BoNT will not enter the neuron at all, or less toxin will enter the neuron than necessary to achieve a clinical result.

2.2.2. Secondary insensitivity

In cases where the BoNT used to work and suddenly became ineffective, we speak of secondary insensitivity. It can be objective or subjective, full or partial, permanent or temporary.

Among its causes are psychological factors; for example, many clinicians have noted a weaker effect when the patient is in a depressive state.

Treatment effectiveness may be insufficient during the exacerbation of an underlying disease, due to an injection technique mistake during the procedure, or owing to reduced drug activity.

Finally, the patient may develop immune resistance to BoNT associated with the formation of neutralizing antibodies. We will discuss this phenomenon in more detail next.

2.2.3. Immune resistance to BoNT

Theoretically, antibodies can be developed to any component of the botulinum toxin complex. After all, they are all peptides, and peptides are known to be the strongest antigens. The question is to which proteins will antibodies be produced (**Fig. I-2-1**) (Bellows S., Jankovic J., 2019).

If antibodies pertain to hemagglutinin, the clinical activity of the drug will be practically unaffected. After its injection into the muscle, rapid dissociation of the complex will occur, the hemagglutinin will leave, and the neurotoxin will take effect (Martin M.U. et al., 2024).

But if antibodies are developed to one of the core neurotoxin chains, the drug activity will decrease (Carr W.W. at al., 2021). Such cases have been described, but they relate to the regular use of BoNT in high doses for neurological indications (Srinoulprasert Y., Wanitphakdeedecha R., 2020).

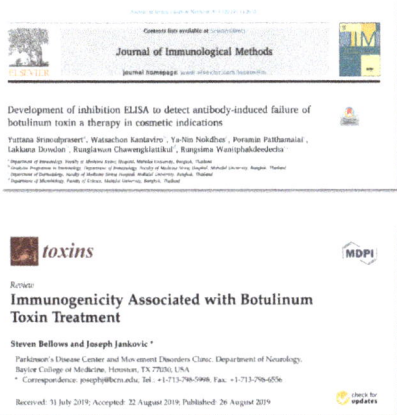

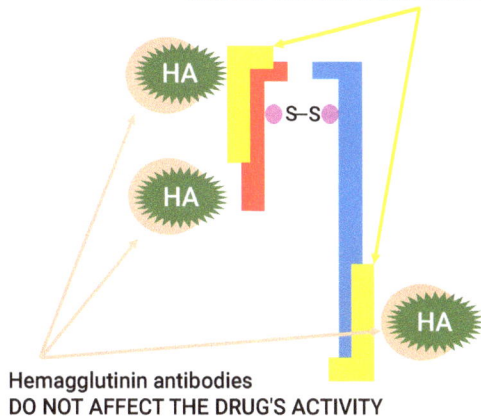

Antibodies to the peptide chains of neurotoxin
REDUCE THE DRUG'S ACTIVITY

Hemagglutinin antibodies
DO NOT AFFECT THE DRUG'S ACTIVITY

Figure I-2-1. Immune resistance to botulinum toxin

This outcome is very rare when the drug is used for aesthetic purposes. Moreover, the risks of immune resistance can be reduced by following these recommendations:

1. Use optimal therapeutic doses of the drug
2. Maintain at least 12-week intervals between treatments
3. Avoid frequent low-dose injections

Immunity to BoNT is unstable, so if secondary insensitivity develops, patients should refrain from injections for at least a year. Once the procedures are resumed, the effect should be as before.

2.3. Adequate assessment of indications and contraindications

Another critical aspect determining the therapy outcome is an adequate assessment of indications (**Fig. I-2-2**) and contraindications (see Part I, section 4.1).

Most people who are not knowledgeable in aesthetic medicine strongly believe that botulinum toxin removes any wrinkle. This is only partially true because it can be used to smooth only those wrinkles

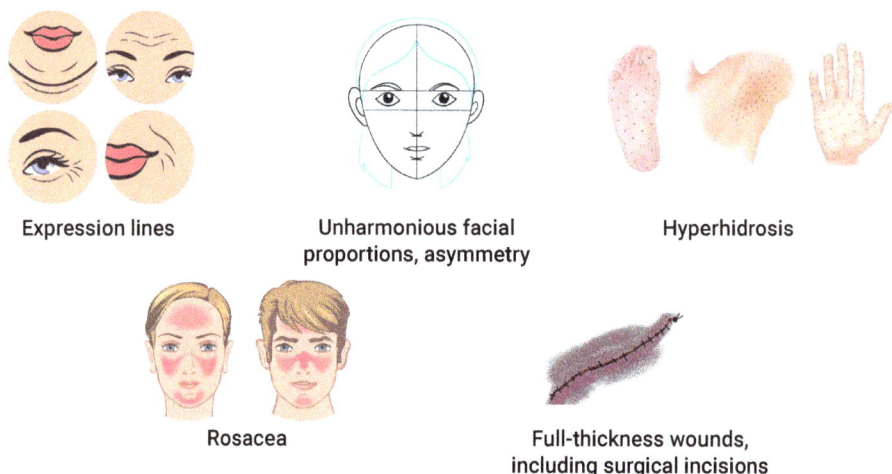

Expression lines

Unharmonious facial proportions, asymmetry

Hyperhidrosis

Rosacea

Full-thickness wounds, including surgical incisions

Figure I-2-2. Primary aesthetic and dermatologic indications for botulinum therapy

that have appeared due to overactive facial expressions or hypertonus of specific muscles (**Fig. I-2-3**). These wrinkles are called **expression lines, mimic wrinkles,** or **dynamic wrinkles**.

Expression lines occur in some anatomical regions and can appear at a relatively young age. By looking at a teenager's face, it is possible to predict the localization of expression lines in the future quite accurately.

However, some wrinkles are associated with age-related changes in the face — skin, subcutaneous tissues, bone skeleton — and with the action of gravity. Such wrinkles are called **static**.

For example, the tear furrow appears due to age-related structural changes in the orbital region. It is corrected with hyaluronic acid-based fillers that compensate for the volume deficit.

Gravity causes "marionette" wrinkles and deepening of the naso-labial fold. In this area, the skin becomes less elastic over time and starts to sag as it can no longer effectively counteract the force of gravity. Some energy-based and injectable methods can tighten it, but if this does not help, surgical lifting or installing a thread frame is necessary.

A grid of fine lines is associated with dryness of the *stratum corneum* — it can be easily removed with moisturizing skincare products.

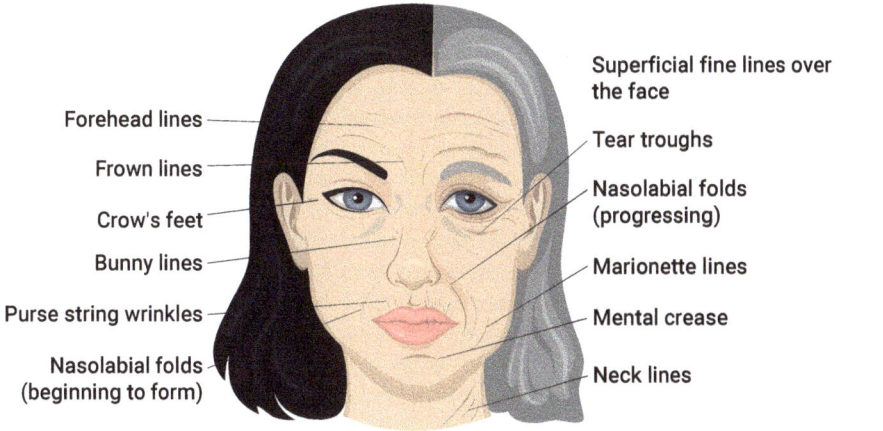

DYNAMIC WRINKLES (EXPRESSION LINES)		STATIC WRINKLES (GRAVITATIONAL, AGE-RELATED)	

Forehead lines
Frown lines
Crow's feet
Bunny lines
Purse string wrinkles
Nasolabial folds (beginning to form)

Superficial fine lines over the face
Tear troughs
Nasolabial folds (progressing)
Marionette lines
Mental crease
Neck lines

Prevention:	Correction:	Prevention:	Correction:
■ Botulinum therapy	■ Botulinum therapy	■ Cosmetic care	■ Fillers
	■ Fillers	■ Mesotherapy	■ Threads
	■ Threads	■ RF lifting	■ Microneedling
		■ Photorejuvenation	■ Fractional RF therapy
			■ Fractional photothermolys
			■ High-intensity focused ultrasound therapy

Figure I-2-3. Types of wrinkles and the aesthetic methods for their prevention and correction

Botulinum therapy is not a one-size-fits-all solution to wrinkles. Sometimes, it will not work and must be combined with other aesthetic treatments for optimal results (see **Fig. I-2-3**).

Nowadays, BoNT is used not only for wrinkle reduction but also for face harmonization. After all, the facial skeleton, the volume of soft tissues, and the muscular framework of the face determine its contours and the mutual arrangement of specific facial components (see Part I, chapter 3).

Today, skincare practitioners are increasingly confronted with skin conditions and pathologies traditionally treated by dermatologists and other specialty physicians. Such conditions include scars due to

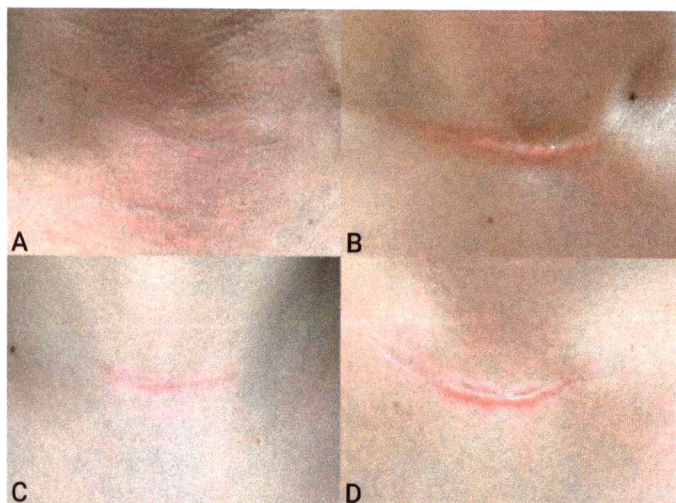

Figure I-2-4. Postoperative scars 24 weeks after open thyroidectomy (adapted from Bae D.S. et al., 2020): (A) a 54-year-old male treated with BoNT microdose injections; (B) a 41-year-old female in the control group (no BoNT treatment); (C) a 46-year-old male treated with BoNT microdose injections; (D) a 54-year-old female in the control group (no BoNT treatment)

full-thickness wounds. The skin may have been traumatized in an accident, or an incision may have been made with a surgical scalpel. Scarring is inevitable if the basal membrane is damaged linearly or over a large area. Injecting the edges of the incision or wound with microdoses of BoNT reduces the activity of myofibroblasts and thereby reduces the tensile force acting on the wound edges. Clinically, this has been shown to promote the healing process and thus results in the formation of a less prominent scar (**Fig. I-2-4**) (Hu L. et al., 2018; Kasyanju Carrero L.M. et al., 2019; Bae D.S. et al., 2020). Recent studies have shed light on the subtle molecular mechanisms of the modulatory effects of BoNT on the process of hypertrophic scar formation by demonstrating a dose-dependent decrease in the mRNA levels of smooth muscle cell alpha-actin and collagen types I and III in fibroblasts pre-stimulated with transforming growth factor beta (TGF-β1) (Li Y.H. et al., 2021).

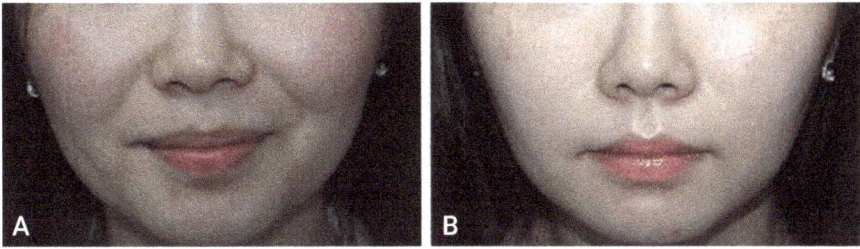

Figure I-2-5. Rosacea: (A) before and (B) eight weeks after intradermal microdose BoNT injections (adapted from Park K.Y. et al., 2018)

Another example is rosacea. Many publications in the medical literature describe successful treatment of this dermatologic disease with intradermal microdose BoNT injections (**Fig. I-2-5**) (Park K.Y. et al., 2018). In particular, BoNT has been shown to block mast cell degranulation, thereby reducing inflammatory response and erythema in patients with rosacea (Choi J.E. et al., 2019).

Medical literature also provides evidence of successful BoNT applications in individuals with oily skin, in whom intradermal microdose BoNT injections reduced sebum production and secretion. The blockade of cholinergic signal transmission from neurons to sebocytes probably underlies this effect (Shuo L. et al., 2019).

Hyperhidrosis, a functional disorder of the sweating system resulting in profuse perspiration, can be treated by BoNT injections. The eccrine sweat glands are under the control of the sympathetic section of the autonomic nervous system. Peripheral regulation of sweating occurs due to cholinergic nerve fibers — sympathetic postganglionic unmyelinated class C fibers that braid the secretory portion of the gland. To meliorate hyperhidrosis, multiple intradermal injections of BoNT are made in sweat gland areas (axillae, palms, feet) to block signal transmission to sweat cells (Nawrocki S., Cha J., 2020). The procedure is painful and requires anesthesia. The clinical effect occurs in the first two days after injections and persists for 6–12 months.

In the next chapter, we will focus on the main objectives of aesthetic botulinum therapy in the face and neck.

Chapter 3
Botulinum therapy in the face and neck

We can distinguish five main categories of aesthetic indications for botulinum therapy in the face and neck.

3.1. Prevention and reduction of dynamic wrinkles

BoNT application in aesthetic medicine began with the correction of expression lines. Initially, it was glabellar and forehead wrinkles, then BoNT started to be used on "crow's feet" in the outside corners of the eyes. Over time, BoNT was introduced into other areas of the face, and today, full-face protocols are actively practiced, involving BoNT injection into different regions in a single procedure, even when forehead wrinkles are the main aesthetic problem (**Fig. I-3-1**) (Kwon K.H. et al., 2019; Nikolis A. et al., 2020).

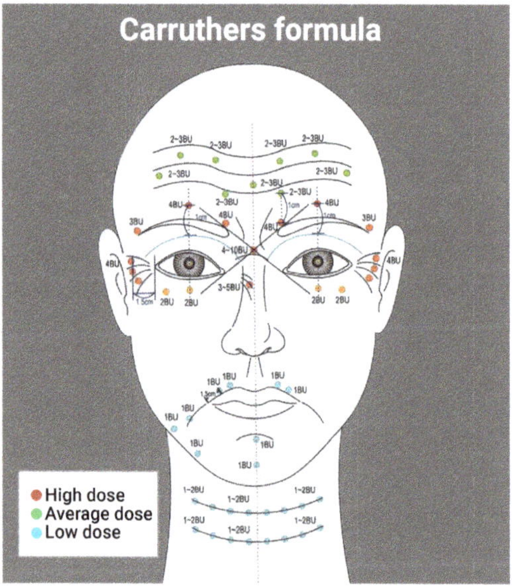

The fact is that the formation of skin folds and expression lines is often determined by the work

Figure I-3-1. BoNT injection points and approximate doses (given in Botox units, BU) for expression line reduction (adapted from Kwon K.H. et al., 2019)

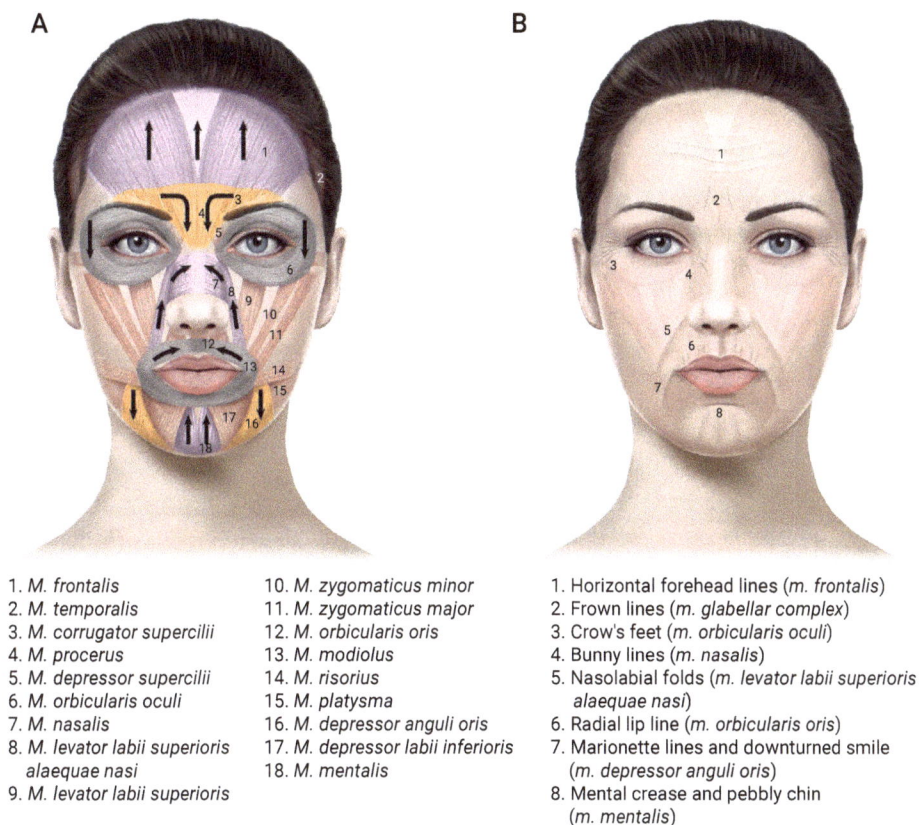

A

B

1. *M. frontalis*
2. *M. temporalis*
3. *M. corrugator supercilii*
4. *M. procerus*
5. *M. depressor supercilii*
6. *M. orbicularis oculi*
7. *M. nasalis*
8. *M. levator labii superioris alaequae nasi*
9. *M. levator labii superioris*
10. *M. zygomaticus minor*
11. *M. zygomaticus major*
12. *M. orbicularis oris*
13. *M. modiolus*
14. *M. risorius*
15. *M. platysma*
16. *M. depressor anguli oris*
17. *M. depressor labii inferioris*
18. *M. mentalis*

1. Horizontal forehead lines (*m. frontalis*)
2. Frown lines (*m. glabellar complex*)
3. Crow's feet (*m. orbicularis oculi*)
4. Bunny lines (*m. nasalis*)
5. Nasolabial folds (*m. levator labii superioris alaequae nasi*)
6. Radial lip line (*m. orbicularis oris*)
7. Marionette lines and downturned smile (*m. depressor anguli oris*)
8. Mental crease and pebbly chin (*m. mentalis*)

Figure I-3-2. (A) Mimic muscles and (B) associated expression lines (adapted from Small R., 2014)

of several facial muscles (**Fig. I-3-2**) (Small R., 2014). Although their contribution is likely to be unequal and one tends to predominate, others should also be considered if a more natural aesthetic result is sought (Flavio A., 2018).

Typically, most wrinkles in the upper half of the face appear after 35 years of age, and those in the lower half start to emerge after 45. Suppose static wrinkles have not yet appeared, and dynamic wrinkles are pronounced during expression. In that case, BoNT injections can delay their appearance (e.g., cicatricial wrinkles of the smoker's upper lip and the lower third of the face and neck).

In some cases, BoNT is used for young patients (about 20 years old) to prevent "crow's feet" formation. While 50% of the patients were previously in the 45–55 age group, and 25–35-year-olds comprised only about 20%, young patients increasingly turn to preventive botulinum therapy (Kattimani V. et al., 2019).

In addition, injecting BoNT into specific areas can help lessen incorrect facial expressions and create a new pattern that harmonizes the face. For example, injecting BoNT between eyebrows can help the patient "unlearn" habitual frowning that involves the masseter muscles or stop clenching the teeth hard when unnecessary.

3.2. Smoothing the skin surface

Superficial intradermal injection of BoNT microdoses does not significantly weaken the tone of the underlying muscles but allows it to affect individual superficial muscle fibers embedded in the skin. This **microdroplet** method can be used to lessen fine wrinkles in areas where intramuscular injection of BoNT is inadmissible (as a rule, we are talking about the zygomatic and cheek areas of the face). After this treatment, the skin relaxes slightly, and wrinkles become less visible (Kandhari R. et al., 2022).

It should be noted that skin quality improves when botulinum treatment is combined with mesotherapy, biorevitalization, or platelet-rich plasma (PRP) therapy (see Part IV, section 2.3).

3.3. Harmonious weakening of the tonus of the whole muscle or its portion

Muscle(s) hypertonus will cause the face to become skewed. Of course, we do not have a completely symmetrical face, and a slight asymmetry adds uniqueness and charm.

But sometimes asymmetry becomes very pronounced and will be considered an aesthetic defect (Kim D. et al., 2020). This can be observed, for example, in facial nerve paresis, when mimic muscles on one side of the face are weakened or even paralyzed. In this case, BoNT injections into the muscles on the opposite side of the face can help restore balance (**Fig. I-3-3**).

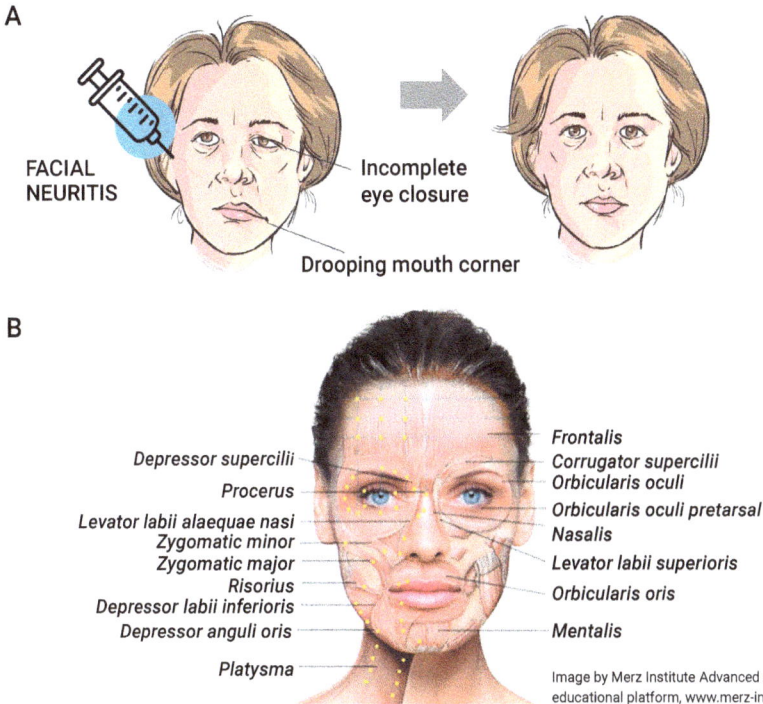

A

FACIAL
NEURITIS

Incomplete
eye closure

Drooping mouth corner

B

Depressor supercilii
Procerus
Levator labii alaequae nasi
Zygomatic minor
Zygomatic major
Risorius
Depressor labii inferioris
Depressor anguli oris

Platysma

Frontalis
Corrugator supercilii
Orbicularis oculi
Orbicularis oculi pretarsal
Nasalis
Levator labii superioris
Orbicularis oris

Mentalis

Image by Merz Institute Advanced Aesthetics
educational platform, www.merz-institute.com

Figure I-3-3. (A) Loosening the muscle on the opposite side with BoNT injection will help restore facial symmetry in cases of severe asymmetry; (B) Possible BoNT injection points in mimic muscles in facial paralysis

3.4. Restoring the balance between agonist and antagonist muscles

The activity of most facial muscles is balanced. The relative position of specific facial components depends on that balance. For example, the position and shape of the eyebrows rely on the state of the frontal levator muscles (*m. frontalis*) which raise the eyebrow, and circular ocular depressor muscles (*m. orbicularis oculi*) that lower the eyebrow (see **Fig. I-3-2A**) (Small R., 2014).

We can apply the same rule to the facial contour, which is determined by the levators (zygomatic muscles, which lift the upper lip) and depressors (muscles that lower the mouth corners and the lower lip, as well as platysma). By weakening the depressors, we "ease" the work of the levators, achieving changes in facial contour.

When performing the procedure, it is extremely important to consider the balance between muscles with multidirectional action and affect them with optimal doses, considering the possibility of the antagonist muscles forming compensatory wrinkles.

3.5. Changes in facial volume and proportions

The volume of dormant muscles decreases quite quickly. This is easy to see in patients with a leg fracture — after the cast is removed, the injured leg is usually much smaller in volume than the healthy leg. As the load increases, the muscle volume is restored.

Mimic muscles are no exception: in the absence of the ability to contract, their volume is also reduced to a greater or lesser extent. This effect has been successfully utilized to treat existing hypertrophy of masticatory muscles: injecting BoNT into these muscles reduces their tone and functional activity (Kwon K.H. et al., 2019; Rauso R. et al., 2021) and, over time, leads to a decrease in their volume (**Fig. I-3-4**).

Similarly, the volume of the glabellar complex muscles also decreases, albeit less noticeably. Over time, in patients who undergo regular glabellar line reduction, this area becomes smoother and bulges less.

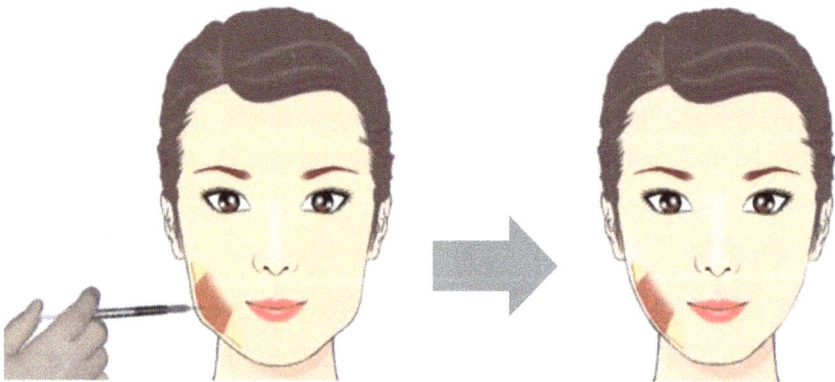

Figure I-3-4. BoNT-assisted treatment of masseter hypertrophy

Chapter 4
Safety of botulinum therapy

4.1. Contraindications to botulinum therapy

Absolute contraindications:

- Myasthenia gravis* and myasthenia gravis-like syndromes — an autoimmune neuromuscular condition characterized by rapid fatigue
- Inflammatory process at the intended injection site
- Acute infectious disease
- Hemophilia
- High myopia
- Keloidal scarring
- Body dysmorphic disorder
- Amyotrophic lateralizing sclerosis myopathies
- General diseases in the stage of exacerbation

Relative contraindications:

- Allergy
- Administration of myorelaxants, anticoagulants, antidepressants, and antibiotics from the group of aminoglycosides, tetracycline, and polymyxin
- Alcohol abuse
- Expressed gravitational ptosis of facial tissues, eyelid hernias
- Facial architectonics features

_____

*Myasthenia gravis is a chronic neuromuscular disease that causes weakness in the voluntary muscles, i.e., those that connect to bones, as well as muscles in the face, throat, and diaphragm. They contract to move the arms and legs and are essential for breathing, swallowing, and facial movements.

- Tendency to facial edema
- Unstable mental state
- Unrealistic patient expectations about treatment outcomes

The current consensus is that the use of BoNT for vital indications during pregnancy and lactation is acceptable but should not be offered for aesthetic reasons (Small R., 2014; Kattimani V. et al., 2019; Padda I.S., Tadi P., 2024).

4.2. Adverse events and complications

If the treatment is performed correctly, the risks of adverse events and complications are MINIMAL!

Accumulated clinical experience shows that complications due to the use of BoNT preparations for aesthetic indications (**Fig. I-4-1**) occur 33 times less frequently than when BoNT is used for medical indications (Walker T.J., Dayan S.H., 2014; Yiannakopoulou E., 2015; Sundaram H. et al., 2016a).

BoNT does not pass through the blood–brain barrier or enter the central nervous system, and it does not pass through the placental barrier either.

COMPLICATIONS ARE RARE AND ALWAYS REVERSIBLE!

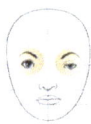

- Excessive weakness of the target muscles and neighboring muscles: drooping of the upper eyelid, speaking difficulties, smile asymmetry, "freezing" of emotions

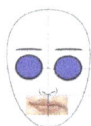

- Puffiness around the eyes: at risk are individuals of the mongoloid race and those who suffer from barley in the eye (hordeolum) and have low periorbital muscle tone

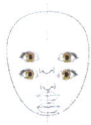

- Appearance of compensatory wrinkles above the eyebrows or at the inner corner of the eyes

- Diplopia (double vision)

Figure I-4-1. Complications associated with BoNT aesthetic injections

When BoNT is used for aesthetic indications, general symptoms such as malaise, nausea, headache, asthenia (chronic fatigue syndrome), and flu-like syndrome may sometimes occur.

Localized symptoms such as pain at the injection site, hemorrhage, and transient hypoesthesia (decreased sensitivity to stimuli) can be expected.

Incorrect injection techniques are also associated with some undesirable effects. For example, inaccurate determination of injection points and dose may lead to excessive weakening of both target and neighboring muscles, upper eyelid drooping, speech difficulties, and inability to express emotions.

Swelling around the eyes may occur, especially in those of mongoloid race, those suffering from hordeolum (stye), and those with low periorbital muscle tone.

The appearance of compensatory wrinkles above the eyebrows or at the inner corners of the eyes is also common. However, correct BoNT injection in the upper third of the face helps avoid this undesirable yet predictable outcome.

On the other hand, many who suffer from migraines notice relief after a BoNT procedure in the upper third of the face. The head, face, and neck muscles can be involved in the development of headaches — if they are overstretched, a person feels pain. BoNT relaxes the muscles, the pain subsides, and the frequency of migraines is reduced. While this effect is unfortunately reversible, tension headaches and migraines are already firmly on the list of indications for the BoNT use (Becker W.J., 2020).

In all the years of BoNT application in aesthetic medicine, there have been no cases of disability or irreversible or lethal complications.

4.3. Some unfounded fears and concerns about botulinum therapy

When done correctly, botulinum therapy is a highly safe procedure. Even if an unexpected unpleasant situation happens, it is always reversible. Nonetheless, many speculations surrounding BoNT are fueled by emotions and misconceptions rather than facts (Dover J.S. et al., 2018).

4.3.1. Can I get botulism after botulinum therapy?

The word "toxin" sounds threatening, causing many to feel afraid about its potential effects on their health.

Indeed, BoNT is a potent poison, but everything depends on the dose. If we make calculations focusing on the activity units of Botox 100, we get the following picture.

The Botox dose that can cause lethal outcomes in 50% of cases is 3000 units. This is equivalent to 30 vials for parenteral administration, bypassing the gastrointestinal tract. When taken orally, the toxic dose is at least 10,000 times higher, and to reach it, you will have to drink the contents of 300,000 vials.

Other drugs have different activity units in absolute figures. Still, the essence of the calculation does not change — the lethal dose of each will be many times higher than the therapeutic dose.

For Botox treatment, the maximal total dose during one session is about 500 units; this amount is not delivered in one but several injections in different areas. Such high-dose procedures can be carried out to treat hyperhidrosis at several locations simultaneously (palm, foot, axillary area, face, and head) or if the patient shows low sensitivity to standard doses. Usually, however, in an aesthetic correction on the face and neck, the total dose of the injected toxin is 5–6 times lower.

Therefore, **the fears that botulinum therapy may cause botulism have no basis. To reduce the negative perception of the method associated with the word "toxin," neurologists have proposed avoiding this word and using the term "botulinum neuroprotein."**

4.3.2. Can botulinum toxin be injected into any muscle?

The use of BoNT in many areas of clinical medicine, including neurology and ophthalmology, where this treatment was first adopted, gynecology, psychiatry, cardiology, dentistry, maxillofacial surgery, etc., indicates that there are no muscles in the body into which BoNT cannot be injected in case of hyperactivity or spasm without jeopardizing health.

In other words, **any transverse striated muscle can be a target for BoNT**.

4.3.3. Can botulinum therapy be given to pregnant women?

Despite the growing evidence regarding BoNT safety, many still believe that botulinum toxin is a poison that it will circulate in the blood for six months, harming the woman and the fetus. In some cases, pregnancy termination is advised if the woman has recently undergone BoNT treatment.

Such misconceptions arise from medical illiteracy but can have negative consequences.

To alleviate these concerns, it is worth noting that, based on the retrospective study conducted by Brin M.F. et al. (2016), botulinum therapy does not lead to an increase in the number of fetal complications, worsening of the course of pregnancy, or an increase in the number of deformities compared to the background rates in the general population (**Fig. I-4-2**). The authors reached these conclusions after analyzing the course of 574 pregnancies. Patients were followed for 24 months (before, during, and after pregnancy).

These findings indicate that **botulinum therapy for medical reasons can be performed during pregnancy**.

Still, BoNT use for aesthetic indications is not advised during pregnancy, not because there is a threat to the child but because during pregnancy, the hormonal background of the female body changes. As a result, the risks of undesirable reactions, including edema, are higher. The priorities of pregnant women are different, so such an unrestrained desire for invasive beauty treatments in any state is more likely to speak of a mental disorder rather than an objective need.

As to whether the toxin is excreted into women's milk, in the absence of large-scale studies involving humans, it is better to abstain from BoNT use while breastfeeding.

4.3.4. Are there age restrictions for botulinum therapy?

Scientific research and considerable practical experience show that there is no age limit to the use of botulinum therapy. With its widespread use in all age groups, it has been successfully performed, for

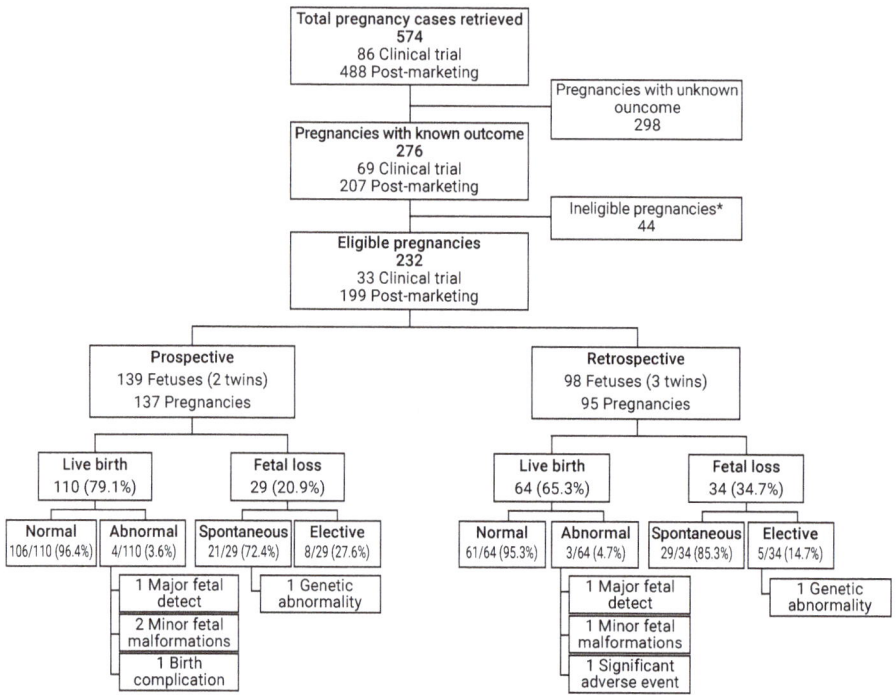

Figure I-4-2. Distribution of pregnancy cases*

example, on newborns with congenital clubfoot, children of all ages with spasticity (Wright E., Fetsko L., 2021), and patients over 90 years of age for both therapeutic and aesthetic purposes.

Indeed, in medicine, there is no alternative to injectable botulinum therapy to pinpoint and precisely relax target muscles for a prolonged period.

In aesthetic medicine, on the other hand, non-injectable products are positioned on the market as "botulinum toxin effect-like," as discussed below.

_____

*Pregnancies in which onabotulinumtoxinA injection occurred > 3 months before the estimated date of conception (adapted from Brin M.F. et al., 2016)

4.3.5. Is there a non-injectable alternative to botulinum therapy?

BoNT cannot be used in cosmetic products.

First, it's illegal, as BoNT is a drug.

Second, it is technically impossible, given that BoNT is highly unstable and rapidly deactivates during cosmetic product manufacture, storage, and application.

Third, BoNT molecule is too large and will not pass through the *stratum corneum*.

Still, reducing the mimic activity to prevent and treat expression lines is tempting. Therefore, cosmetic chemists, almost simultaneously with the appearance of botulinum toxin in the aesthetic field, began to search for an alternative. As a result of these efforts, in 2003, a new category of cosmetics appeared on the market — products "with the effect of botulinum toxin." Active ingredients in these preparations are **synthetic peptides** capable of blocking signal transmission from the nerve endings to the muscle fiber. That's why they are called **"Botox-like"** (see Part V, section 1.1).

Argireline® (name according to the International Nomenclature of Cosmetic Ingredients — INCI: Acetyl Hexapeptide-8) was the first peptide in this group to be discovered. Still, others soon followed and there are about 20 currently on the market. They have nothing in common with botulinum toxin in their origin and structure. Their molecular mechanism of action at the synapse level is also different, but the result — muscle relaxation — is similar. This is true, but there is one caveat: the relaxation effect is observed in cell cultures when the peptide is added directly to the cell culture medium. In reality, the peptide has to pass through the *stratum corneum* and reach the muscle in the right amount, and this is problematic. Therefore, in the case of cosmetics with "Botox-like" peptides, we cannot talk about a predictable dose-dependent effect of target muscle relaxation, and it will not happen. The maximum that can be expected from such products is to maintain the effect of injectable botulinum therapy.

Topical BoNT technology, which includes modified neurotoxin in ta cosmetic composition, is an exception to this rule. "Botox-like" peptides and topical BoNT will be discussed more in Part V, section 1.2.

Résumé

To conclude this section, let's list the most important things to remember about botulinum therapy:

1. **BoNT is a naturally occurring, potent poison with nerve agent action.** It blocks the signal transmission from the nerve endings to the muscle or sweat cell. As a result, the muscle remains relaxed, and the sweat cells do not produce sweat.
2. **BoNT is a drug.** Only registered preparations should be used while ensuring that they have been transported and stored under special carefully controlled conditions.
3. **BoNT is used in many areas of medicine when muscles need to be relaxed.** Any muscle of the body can be a target for BoNT.
4. **Botulinum therapy is a safe method with minimal adverse reactions and complication risks.**
   - The action of BoNT is reversible as innervation is restored.
   - The doses used for medical and even more so for aesthetic reasons are hundreds of times lower than the lethal amounts.
   - BoNT does not pass through the blood–brain barrier and does not affect the central nervous system.
   - BoNT does not pass through the placental barrier and does not affect the fetus.
   - There are no age restrictions for the BoNT application.
5. **Botulinum toxin injection requires good anatomical knowledge.** Only physicians with specialized training are allowed to perform this procedure.
6. **There is currently no suitable alternative to injectable botulinum therapy**, although the search in this direction is expected to continue until this goal is attained. This includes developing cosmetic products "with the effect of botulinum toxin" as they can improve skin quality, including wrinkle smoothing. Still, their action mechanisms differ from those of BoNT, and a predictable dose-dependent relaxing effect on the target is absent.

Part II

The paradoxes of aesthetic botulinum therapy

Due to the rapid and beneficial visual effects, minimal invasiveness, and simplicity of the procedure, botulinum therapy remains one of the most popular aesthetic treatments. According to the American Society of Plastic Surgeons (ASPS), BoNT/A aesthetic injections are firmly in the lead among non-surgical aesthetic procedures (www.plasticsurgery.org). As a result, not only is aesthetic botulinum therapy actively developing as an independent field, but indications for BoNT application are also expanding, new methodological recommendations are being developed, injection techniques are being modified, and doses are evolving. All this ensures optimization of the results achieved, increasing patient satisfaction.

The views on the essence of botulinum therapy are also gradually changing. Whereas we previously considered it solely as an effective way to temporarily eliminate wrinkles in active expression areas of the face, we are now increasingly talking about a global method of aesthetic geroprotection, as well as prevention of facial aging at the level of not only muscles but also skin, ligamentous apparatus, and facial fat (Le Louarn C., 2009a, 2024).

The growing popularity of botulinum therapy has led to the formation of a rather large cohort of patients who have been regularly treated with BoNT/A injections for several years, and such procedures are planned in the future. That is why, in our opinion, it is essential to analyze the possible impact of prolonged BoNT/A exposure on the morphology and physiology of facial muscles, and potentially on the psychology of patients, as well as the expression stereotypes of emotional response.

In practice, BoNT/A therapy is always performed considering the individual features of expression and the mimic muscle anatomy, aiming

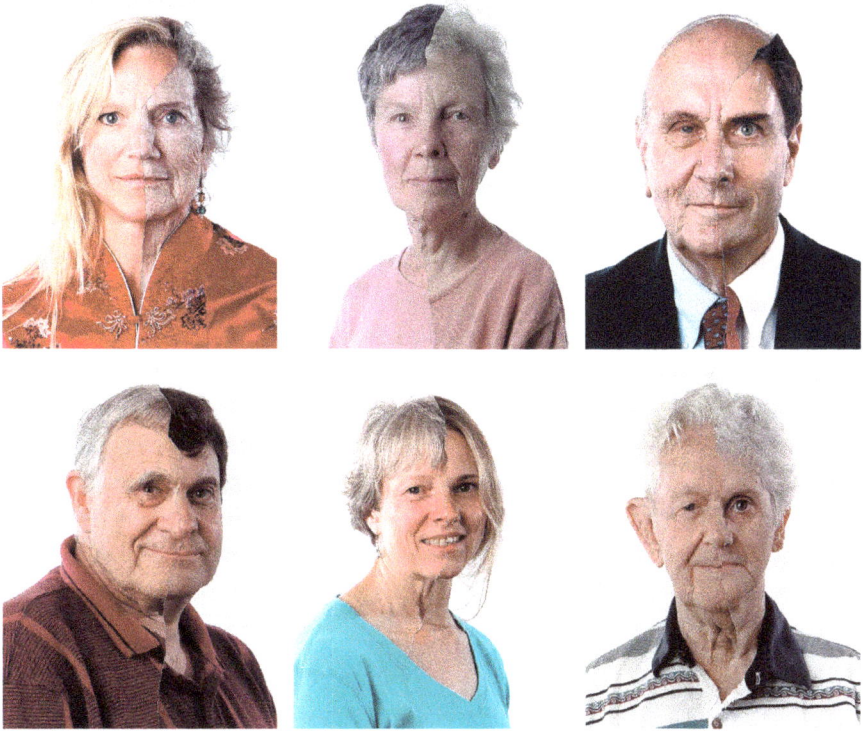

Figure II-1. AgeMaps Photo Project by Bobby Neel Adams
(https://www.bobbyneeladams.com)

to attain the clinical picture of involutional changes. Facial aging features are likely genetically predetermined, including particular morphotypes, given that different generations of the same family exhibit similarity in the rate and character of involutional changes in subcutaneous fat deposits and the patterns of expression. Many practitioners have noticed this phenomenon when observing a mother and her daughter simultaneously. It is thus not uncommon for a physician to ask a patient to bring a recent photograph of her mother before planning a rejuvenation program.

The American photographer Bobby Neel Adams demonstrated the inheritance of the leading facial aging patterns in his AgeMaps photoproject (**Fig. II-1**). He created a series of combined portraits of immediate family members, with one half taken from an image of a mom/dad and the other half representing a daughter/son. As a result, we see not just a "before and now" style snapshot of one person but combined images of two generations at the exact moment in time. If we analyze the photos of parents and their adult children, external similarity, general aging patterns, and the peculiarities of the "pattern" of expression wrinkles can be traced across the generations. Thus, knowing the nature of involutional changes in the parent, we can predict the facial aging of their offspring and build an effective long-term prevention strategy. What role does botulinum therapy play in this approach?

Chapter 1
Positive effects of long-term botulinum therapy

Many patients, having once decided on botulinum toxin injections, become ardent adherents of the method for many years. The accumulated clinical experience testifies to the safety of long-term use of BoNT/A and the preservation of sensitivity to such treatment even with repeated injections (Rzany B. et al., 2007; Dailey R.A. et al., 2011). Using electromyography and facial nerve fiber conduction studies, Devlikamova F.I. et al. (2011) demonstrated that, despite the presence of minimal changes in the muscles of 36 patients who received multiple BoNT/A injections into the mimic muscles of the upper face, botulinum therapy is safe in the long term and does not lead to clinically significant changes in the neuromotor apparatus and the mimic muscles themselves.

The changes produced by the chemical denervation of mimic muscles are multifaceted and extend beyond mere relaxation. The positive effects of BoNT/A injections, including multiple injections, include the following:

- Prevention of expression line formation
- Changes in the skin quality characteristics
- Prevention of early structural aging of the face
- Positive change in facial expression patterns
- Lifting by activating the levator muscles
- Elimination of depressor stereotypic expression activity
- Changes in the volume of facial muscles
- Indirect influence on the emotional background

1.1. Reducing expression lines

Leveling skin relief in expression lines is botulinum therapy's direct and most obvious positive effect. Chemical denervation causes a rather prolonged but reversible relaxation of mimic muscles and eliminates their hyperkinetic activity. This effect is most evident when injecting BoNT/A for classical indications to eliminate wrinkles in the forehead (horizontal forehead lines), interbrow area (glabellar lines), and lateral corners of the eyes ("crow's feet"). Long-term BoNT/A use for this indication demonstrates the prophylactic effect of the toxin against wrinkle formation in areas of increased expression activity (Yi K.H. et al., 2022; Yi K.H. et al., 2024).

It is not easy to assess the contribution — either positive or negative — of any particular factor to the character of facial aging in each patient. Therefore, studies conducted among pairs of identical twins are beneficial for this purpose, as we can assume similarity in the clinical picture of age-related changes, provided that there are no significant differences in lifestyle. In most cases, such studies concern the effects of smoking or insolation on skin condition (Martires K.J. et al., 2009; Okada H.C. et al., 2013). However, very few medical studies evaluate the effects of BoNT/A. Indeed, we came across only two articles about two twin sisters, one of whom has had regular botulinum treatments for years to correct wrinkles in the upper third of the face, while the other has had them only a couple of times (Binder W.J., 2006; Rivkin A., Binder W.J., 2015). When comparing the photos, it is evident that the sister who regularly receives BoNT/A injections has almost imperceptible facial wrinkles in the forehead, glabella, and crow's feet area at rest, whereas the other sister has distinct wrinkles. Their expression activity follows the same trend — the regular botulinum therapy user looks younger and has much better facial skin quality (porosity, microrelief, etc.).

However, can we attribute this effect specifically to botulinum therapy? Japanese researchers have analyzed the degree of expression of static and dynamic wrinkles in different areas of the face depending on age, zone, and expression activity (Fujimura T., Hotta M., 2012). They found that **muscle activity is the main cause of wrinkle formation in areas of expression, and wrinkles observed during expression are a predictor of deep wrinkles that persist at rest**.

1.2. Changing skin quality

Some authors believe botulinum therapy's role in facial aesthetic correction is limited solely to muscle relaxation and skin relief smoothing (Cohen-Letessier A., 2009). Others argue that long-term chemodenervation of muscles can lead to their atrophy and deterioration in skin quality due to a decrease in the level of mechanical deformation and physical stimulation of fibroblasts.

Are these fears justified? Numerous studies have proven them wrong.

For example, Bowler P.J. (2008) presented data on a 50-year-old man and a 53-year-old woman who have had regular BoNT/A injections in the interbrow, periorbital, and frontal areas for seven years. The woman received 24 treatments at 4-month intervals, while the man received 21 treatments at 3–6-month intervals. Both patients reported a high level of satisfaction with the results. The author noted qualitative skin improvements over time with the absence of new wrinkles and suggested possible remodeling of the epidermis and dermis at BoNT/A injection sites.

In a pilot study conducted by Chang S.P. et al. (2008), intradermal BoNT/A injection at low doses in the middle and lower thirds of the face was shown to smooth the skin and reduce wrinkle severity without asignificant lifting effect or impact on facial expression.

Possible mechanisms of direct and indirect effects of BoNT/A on the skin may be related to its ability to inhibit inflammatory processes and sebum production (Dayan S.H. et al., 2012; Rose A.E., Goldberg D.J., 2013). In an experimental study, Abdallah Hajj Hussein I. et al. (2012) showed that botulinum toxin accelerates wound healing.

According to Oh S.H. et al. (2012), BoNT/A does not affect the proliferation of fibroblasts in culture and has no toxic effect, but promotes the expression of type I collagen and inhibits the synthesis of matrix metalloproteinases (MMPs).

These effects may manifest following intradermal and subcutaneous BoNT/A injections. However, the creation of relative expression rest in the areas of the face with hyperfunctional wrinkles also provides aging prevention by reducing excessive mechanical load and unphysiological disturbance of relief due to a chronic increase in muscle tone.

1.3. Preventing age-related facial structure changes

Based on his analysis of facial aging patterns and age-related changes in mimic muscles, French plastic surgeon Dr. Claude Le Louarn formulated a new concept of aging called Face Recurve (Le Louarn S. et al., 2007a). Within this framework, Le Louarn considers botulinum therapy as an effective method for preventing wrinkles in the skin and structural aging of the face associated with the redistribution of fat tissue and involutional changes in bone structures. Prophylactic BoNT/A injections reduce the tone of facial muscles without a pronounced disruption of their contractile ability and markedly affect facial expressions.

According to Le Louarn, age-related changes in mimic muscles contribute significantly to overall facial aging. The dynamics of these changes are not yet fully understood and appear to be driven by a more complex process than previously imagined. At a Radiological Society of North America (RSNA) training course in 2010, Okuda I. (2010) presented computer tomography (CT) images of the facial soft tissue of women of different ages (**Fig. II-1-1**). When analyzing the images, it became evident that the main mimic muscles in young people have a curved shape. They flatten under dynamic tension, with axillary adipose tissue pushing upward. With age, the thickness of deep adipose tissue in the active mimic zones decreases while the adipose tissue located under the skin increases, with the muscles becoming flatter at rest.

Thus, in young people, the facial muscles are longer, have a low resting tone, and a large contraction amplitude. The facial muscles are shorter in older people, and their resting tension is higher. Based on these observations, Le Louarn suggested that hypertonicity of the mimic muscles at rest and age-related decrease in the amplitude of their contraction lead to the protrusion of axillary adipose tissue into the subcutaneous layer, the thickness of which increases (Le Louarn C., 2009b). Subsequently, the superficial adipose tissue may be displaced downward, which causes characteristic age-related changes in the lower face.

This hypothesis was partially confirmed by Owsley J.Q. and Roberts C.L. (2008), who analyzed histological data and magnetic resonance imaging (MRI) scans of soft tissues of the middle third of the face. They showed that repetitive contractions of the muscle that

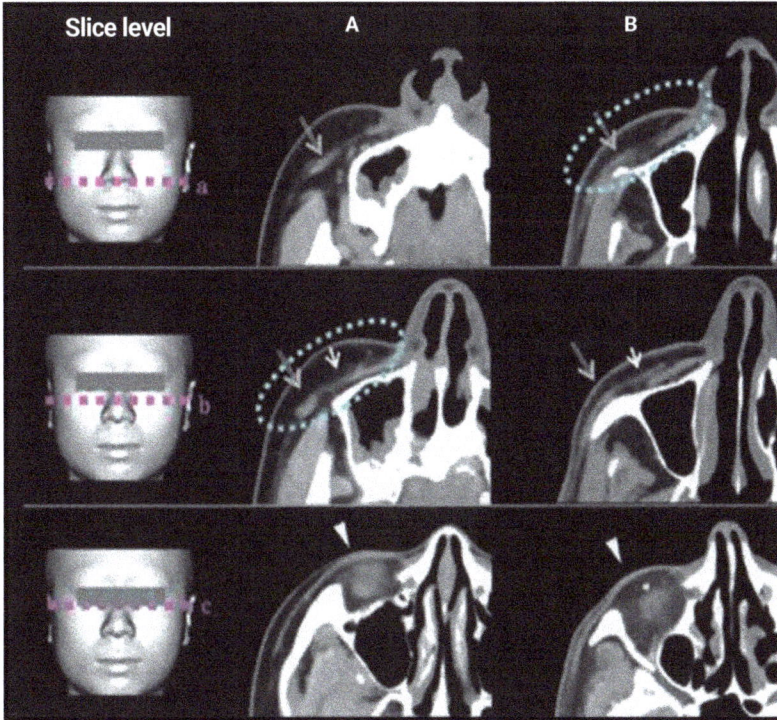

Figure II-1-1. Multilevel CT scans of the face of (A) a 20-year-old and (B) a 78-year-old woman (adapted from Okuda I., 2010)

Long arrows indicate the large zygomatic muscles, and short arrows denote the small ones. Age-related atrophy of these muscles is noted. Due to the increased muscle tone at rest, the axillary adipose tissue is partially pushed upwards during aging, which results in age-related defects in the facial macrorelief. Under the influence of gravity, the adipose tissue (malar fat compartments) is displaced downward (areas marked with blue dotted ovals). Atrophy and increased tone of the circular eye muscle in the lower eyelid area cause the formation of bags under the eyes (indicated by arrows in the lower photos).

lifts the upper lip can lead to a downward displacement of the superficial fat pockets in the cheeks.

Le Louarn also suggested that, even within a single muscle, age-related changes occur in a heterogeneous manner: separate bundles appear — they are so-called age marker fascicles (AMF) — which are significantly shorter than other bundles of the same muscle (serving as evidence of their increased tone), and they are responsible for the structural aging of the face associated with the redistribution of adipose tissue (Le Louarn C., 2009b).

It is also interesting to note that 75 years ago, Mikhail M. Gerasimov, a famous anthropologist and author of the method of facial reconstruction from the skull, wrote: "...deep wrinkles leave their trace in all the underlying soft tissues, and their relief is noticeable even on the bone basis" (Gerasimov M.M., 1949). In other words, dystrophic changes provoked by persistent muscle hypertonus affect the function and structure of the soft tissues and the underlying bones. In this context, **botulinum therapy can be considered as an etiopathogenetic method for preventing structural age-related facial changes by creating a zone of relative "mimic rest."**

1.4. Lifting

BoNT/A lifting is based on the antagonistic interaction of the levator and depressor muscles. Accordingly, the lifting effect can be realized by affecting both levators and depressors.

1.4.1. Working with levators

This mechanism is applicable for eyebrow lifting. In this case, the frontalis muscle is the "target" muscle into which BoNT/A is injected. When the medial portion of the frontalis muscle relaxes, the tone of its inferolateral portion increases in a compensatory manner, achieving the effect of eyebrow lifting.

A similar mechanism operates in correcting the nasolabial fold, which is accentuated by soft tissue overhang. Sometimes, this defect is associated with increased activity of the muscle that lifts the upper lip and wing of the nose. BoNT/A injection into this muscle smooths the nasolabial fold.

1.4.2. Working with depressors

By blocking the depressor muscles in the middle and lower third of the face, which have a centrifugal direction of the contraction vector, we facilitate the work of the levators, which act in the opposite (centripetal) direction. Relaxation of the depressor muscles not only facilitates the work of the levators, but also leads to their dominance:

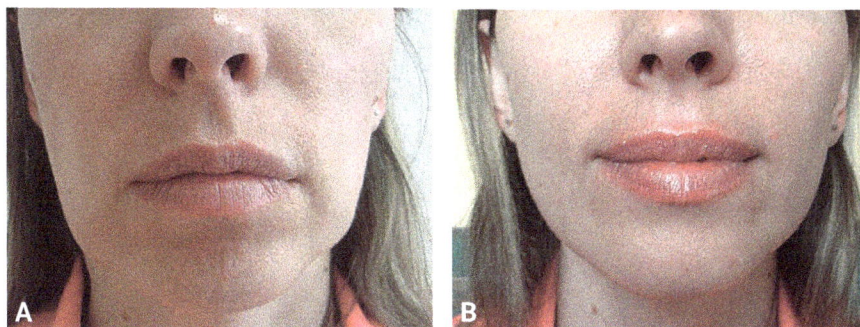

Figure II-1-2. Increase in the volume of the middle third of the face due to the contraction of the zygomatic muscles with the elimination of the activity of the depressor muscles of the lower third of the face (adapted from Sharova A.A., Saromytskaya A.N., 2014)

in the absence of an opposing force, they begin to work more actively and shorten in length, thus producing tissue traction (**Fig. II-1-2**).

The most successful relaxation of the depressor muscles is performed in the middle and lower thirds of the face. However, such manipulations are also possible in the upper third of the face. To achieve a brow lift, injections into the frontalis muscle are often supplemented with small doses of BoNT/A injected into the upper-lateral portion of the circular eye muscle, which is known to be a depressor of the middle and lateral parts of the eyebrow. BoNT/A injections into the muscle that lowers the eyebrow increase the effectiveness of eyebrow lifting, especially of its medial portion (Cook B.E. et al., 2001).

Loss of facial contour definition is associated not only with gravitational ptosis of soft tissues and redistribution of adipose tissue but also with age-related increase in the tone and activity of the depressor muscles of the lower third of the face. Hypertonus of the muscle lowering the corner of the mouth (*m. depressor anguli oris*; DAO) and the platysma can lead to the formation of "grief folds" and "marionette" wrinkles even in young patients. Carruthers J. and Carruthers A. (2001) were the first to report on the possibility of correcting drooping mouth corners by injecting BoNT/A directly into the DAO. In cases where the depressor muscles make a significant contribution to the disfiguration of the facial oval, the use of BoNT/A makes it possible to achieve a noticeable aesthetic effect precisely by redistributing muscle activity between

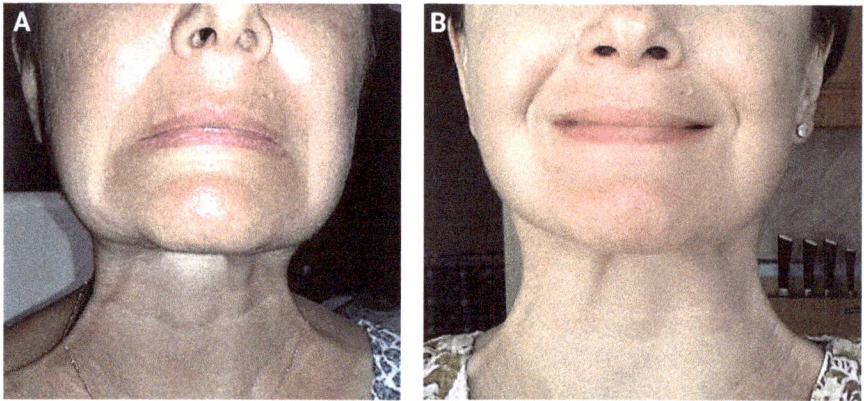

Figure II-1-3. Nefertiti lift is based on the redistribution of muscle activity between the depressors of the lower third of the face and the levators of the middle third (adapted from Sharova A.A., Saromytskaya A.N., 2014)

the depressors of the lower third and the levators of the middle third of the face (**Fig. II-1-3**). The Nefertiti lift, developed by Swiss dermatologist Philippe Levy, is based on this mechanism (Levy P.M., 2007).

Since, in this case, the lifting effect depends solely on the ability of the facial muscles to contract — shifting upward the overlying soft tissues — the crucial conditions for the success of the procedure are:

- Gravitational ptosis of mild (grade 1: up to 2 mm) and moderate (grade 2: 2–3 mm) severity (Quatela V.C., Ahmedli N.N., 2021)
- Thin to medium-thick skin
- Slight to moderate subcutaneous adipose tissue thickness
- Small to medium soft tissue mobility amplitude
- Hyperactivity/hypertension of the depressor muscles of the lower third of the face

In our experience, the most pronounced effect of BoNT/A-assisted lifting is observed in patients aged 35–45. Later, the procedure effectiveness decreases in the same patients, probably due to the increasing displacement of tissues against the background of reducing skin elasticity and ligamentous apparatus, increasing the degree of gravitational ptosis.

1.5. Volumetric transformation of muscles

Using BoNT/A to change muscle volume is another aim of aesthetic botulinum therapy. For this purpose, injections are performed in the masticatory muscles for their hypertrophy in European patients and to correct a square face with normotrophy of the masticatory muscles in Asian patients.

In Europeans, masticatory hypertrophy is commonly associated with bruxism or orthodontic disorders. After botulinum therapy, individuals prone to bruxism notice not only a resolution of the underlying problem, but also an improvement in the shape of their face, which becomes more oval (**Fig. II-1-4**) (Aydil B. et al., 2012). Muscle volume

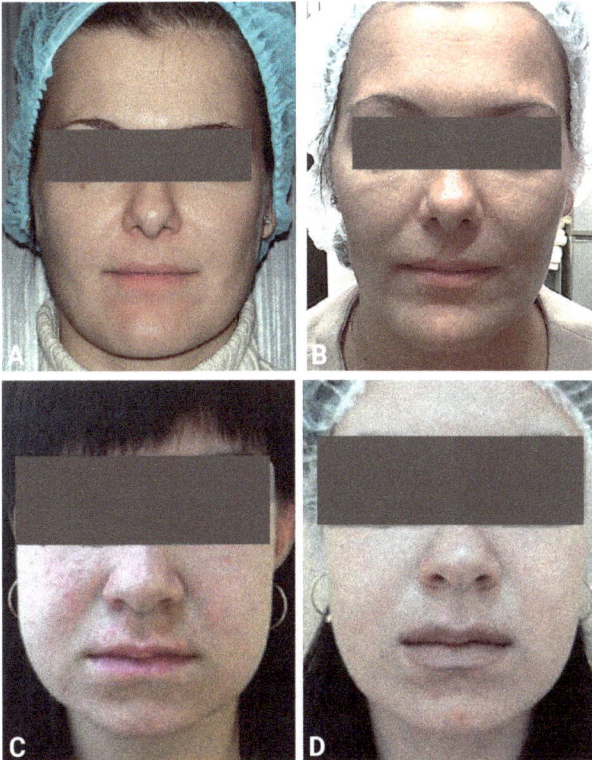

Figure II-1-4. Reduction of facial width in the lower third of the face after multiple BoNT/A injections into the masseter muscles (devolumizing effect) (adapted from Sharova A.A., Saromytskaya A.N., 2014)

reduction occurs due to its hypotrophy against the background of reduced motor activity. This process develops gradually, and its results are noticeable 2–4 weeks after BoNT/A injections. Laser scanning allows the reduction in the volume and width of masticatory muscles after botulinum therapy to be confirmed objectively (Shim W.H. et al., 2010). After 10–12 months, the muscle volume is restored, i.e., the hypotrophy effect is reversible (Ahn K.Y., 2010).

Available evidence also shows that relaxation of mimic muscles, such as those in the interbrow area, also reduces their volume. Such an effect was demonstrated in a study by specialists of the Institute of Clinical Radiology of Ludwig-Maximilian University using MRI findings. After a single BoNT/A injection, a 46−48% decrease in the procerus volume was observed, and this effect persisted for 12 months (Koerte I.K. et al., 2013). Perhaps the observed effect is not related to hypotrophy of the mimic muscle but to a change in its volumetric configuration and shape from flattened when tense to more extended and convex when relaxed, which may appear as a volume reduction on MRI images. Visually, this effect is often observed in patients with large and powerful muscles of the interbrow area that, having increased tone, form a "heavy," convex, folded glabella. In such patients, after several consecutive BoNT/A injections, wrinkles in this area become smoother, and a volume reduction becomes readily apparent, possibly due to the contour smoothing (**Fig. II-1-5**).

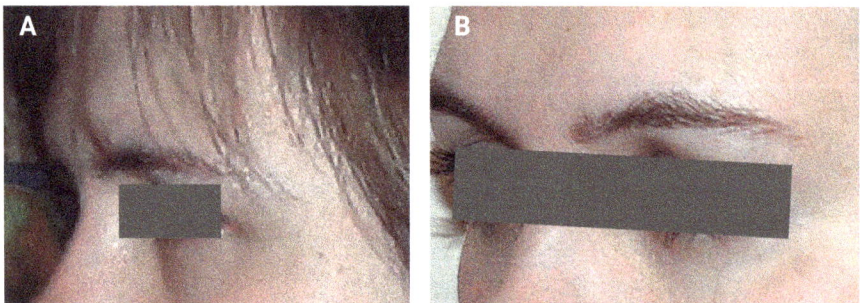

Figure II-1-5. When BoNT/A is regularly injected into the glabella muscles for several years, not only wrinkle smoothing but also volume reduction in this area can be observed (adapted from Sharova A.A., Saromytskaya A.N., 2014)

1.6. Eliminating negative expression stereotypes

In aesthetic medicine, it is customary to classify patients into one or another expression type, which determines the functional state of facial muscles at rest and in dynamics (de Maio M., 2008). Belonging to a particular expression type indicates the prevalence of one or a different kind of expression stereotypy, as the same patient may have a normal tone or even hypotonicity of some muscle groups and hypertonicity of others. In clinical practice, it is thus often necessary to observe hyperkinetic or hypertonic-type patients. In the first case, pathological habits of squinting, frowning, straining the muscles that lower mouth corners, and platysma when forming a skeptical facial expression are often detected. In the second case, even at rest, the face has a frowning, tense expression due to the increased tone of the interbrow muscles, resulting in deep wrinkles.

Patients often also have hypertonicity and/or hyperkinesis of the depressor muscles in the facial lower third. This may result from depressor facial stereotypy or an age-related increase in the activity of these depressor muscles. By eliminating excessive activity of the lower-third depressor muscles and interbrow muscles, it is possible to influence expression stereotypes, creating a more harmonious and positive facial expression. It is also interesting to note that patients often experience a change in the expression line patterns during long-term botulinum therapy (**Fig. II-1-6**).

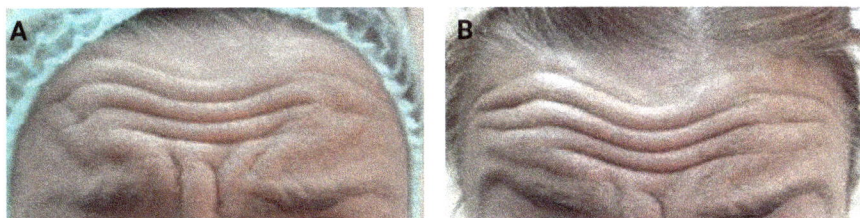

Figure II-1-6. BoNT/A injections for 3 years at 6-month intervals eliminated forehead and glabellar muscle complex coactivity and converted Ω-pattern to V-pattern: (A) before and (B) after treatment (adapted from Sharova A.A., Saromytskaya A.N., 2014)

1.7. Indirect positive influence on the emotional state

Many physicians and patients have noted the effect of botulinum therapy on the person's emotional state. Possible mechanisms of such influence are based on the Facial Feedback Hypothesis principles, formulated by Sylvan Tomkins in 1962 based on the James–Lange theory of emotion (Tomkins S.S., 1981). According to this theory, any emotional experience is amplified and fed by nerve signals from activated facial muscles involved in the facial expression of a given emotion.

Based on the facial feedback hypothesis, Alam M. et al. (2008) analyzed the psychological effects of botulinum therapy. They concluded that modulating the activity of certain mimic muscles can significantly affect the emotional state. Restriction of motor and tonic activity of depressors (especially of the interbrow area) does not block emotions, including negative ones, but weakens their expression.

It has also been established that a person's emotional state and mood are directly related to self-esteem. Visible improvement in appearance with BoNT/A injections in the form of the elimination of expression lines and a more positive facial expression increases self-esteem and, therefore, improves well-being (Costa A.C.F. et al., 2022).

Research into the effects of botulinum therapy on a person's emotional state has prompted several specialists to attempt to use BoNT/A to treat depression. According to a small pilot study on the use of BoNT/A in 10 patients with therapy-resistant depression published in 2006, most of these individuals reported symptom disappearance after BoNT/A injections into the muscles of the interbrow area (Finzi E., Wasserman E., 2006). Even at 18-month follow-up, these effects persisted and were attributed to the periodic BoNT/A injections (Finzi E., 2023).

Even more convincing results of BoNT/A use in the treatment of depression were provided by electromyographic studies, indicating that patients suffering from depression have hyperactive muscles of the interbrow area (Han C. et al., 2012). A randomized placebo-controlled clinical trial conducted by Wollmer M.A. et al. (2012) confirmed the effectiveness of botulinum therapy in such patients: after one BoNT/A injection there was an improvement in well-being, and positive changes were maintained for a year.

Chapter 2
The other side of the coin: "side" effects of aesthetic botulinum therapy

In addition to the positive aspects of BoNT/A preparations in aesthetic facial correction, there are also conditionally "negative" effects — i.e., they are negative exclusively from the aesthetic point of view, not from the medical perspective. These effects are not always apparent, but as we accumulate experience working with patients receiving botulinum therapy for many years, we begin to pay attention to them.

The "negative" effects of long-term botulinum therapy include:

- Appearance of new expression lines or intensification of existing wrinkles
- Formation of compensatory mechanisms associated with the activation of antagonist muscles, additional muscles, or separate portions within one muscle
- Changing facial expression patterns
- Changing the type of emotional response

2.1. Wrinkle appearance or aggravation

The paradoxical effects of long-term BoNT/A use include the appearance of new wrinkles or increased severity of the existing wrinkles that have not been corrected.

When BoNT/A is injected under the tail of the eyebrows to elevate this area, we tend observe the appearance of small horizontal wrinkles above the lateral portion of the eyebrows. This effect seems to be due to tonic activation of the inferior portion of the frontalis muscle, which is embedded in the eyebrow skin. This effect is almost inevitable with a suitable lifting response to botulinum therapy (**Fig. II-2-1**).

In some cases, correction of forehead wrinkles in combination with an attempted BoNT/A brow lift may result in a redistribution of wrinkles: wrinkles in the upper half of the forehead are smoothed out, but a low-lying wrinkle above the brow appears (**Fig. II-2-2**). This wrinkle is challenging to correct, as attempts to inject BoNT/A closer to the new wrinkle either fail (in the case of microdoses of toxin

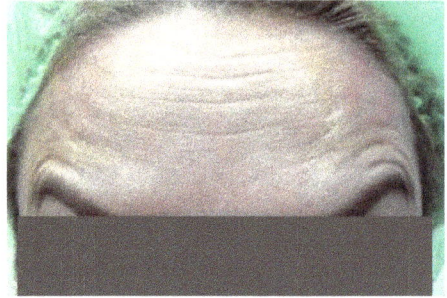

Figure II-2-1. Compensatory wrinkles above the eyebrows with excessive activity of the lateral portion of the frontalis muscles (adapted from Sharova A.A., Saromytskaya A.N., 2014)

and intradermal injection) or result in eyebrow lowering. In the lower third of the face, an increase in the horizontal crease on the chin may be noted in some patients due to the activation of the chin muscle when BoNT/A is injected in the facial oval without correcting the chin muscle.

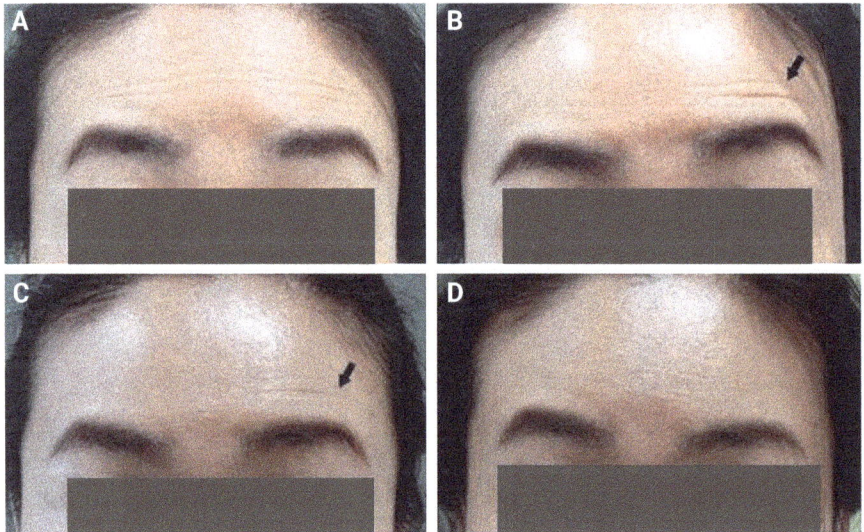

Figure II-2-2. Appearance of new low brow wrinkles: (A) initial picture, (B) one week, (C) two weeks, and (D) four weeks after BoNT/A injections into the frontalis muscle (adapted from Kang S.M. et al., 2011)

Only a few reports of such consequences of aesthetic botulinum therapy have been published. In one of these articles, Kang S.M. et al. (2011) described the appearance of a noticeable bulging of the interbrow area in two patients and the formation of deep unilateral wrinkles just above the eyebrows in two others who had received BoNT/A injection. The authors posited that these effects resulted from the hyperactivity and hypertonus of intact glabellar muscles after isolated correction of the frontal region. This pattern sometimes appears even after a single BoNT/A application and, if ignored, it will only intensify in the future (**Fig. II-2-3**). The primary preventive measure is the combined correction of the frontal and interbrow areas.

2.2. Compensatory mechanisms

Antagonistic muscle interactions must be considered when planning a BoNT/A injection regimen. Underestimation of reciprocal relationships (functional reciprocity) can lead to activating antagonist muscles,

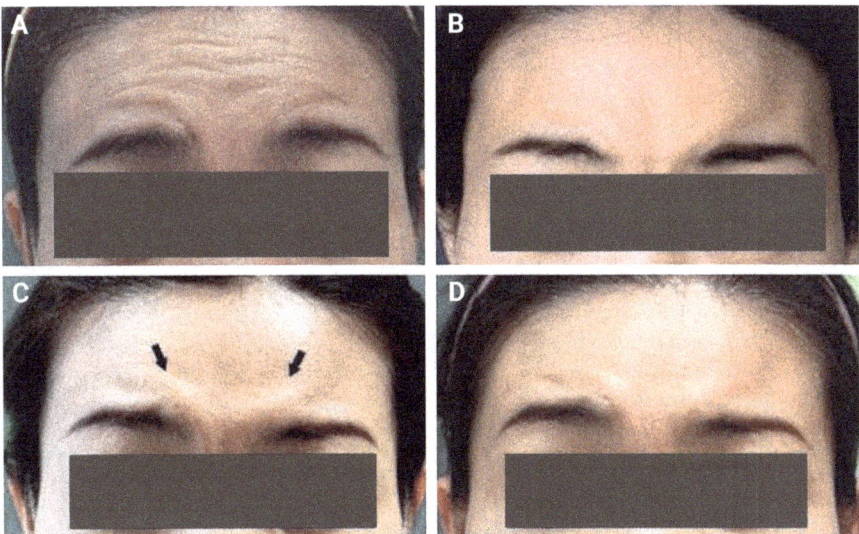

Figure II-2-3. Glabella contouring after BoNT/A injections in the forehead area: (A) patient before treatment at maximum forehead tension, (B) one week, (C) four weeks, and (D) 16 weeks after injections (adapted from Kang S.M. et al., 2011)

additional muscles, or individual portions within the same muscle that were inactive before botulinum toxin correction (**Fig. II-2-4 – II-2-6**).

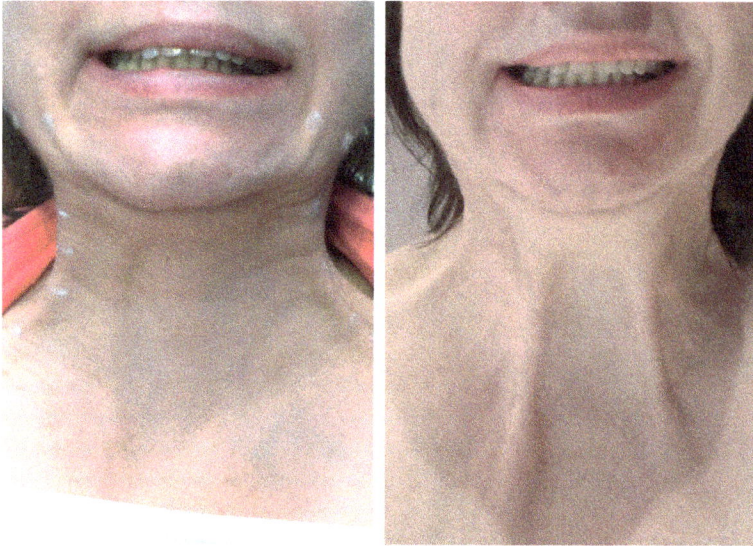

Figure II-2-4. Redistribution of activity within one muscle — platysma (adapted from Sharova A.A., Saromytskaya A.N., 2014)

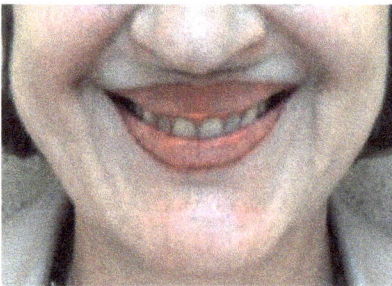

Figure II-2-5. Activation of antagonist muscles: activation of the nasal septum muscle during smiling after isolated correction of the oral circular muscle (adapted from Sharova A.A., Saromytskaya A.N., 2014)

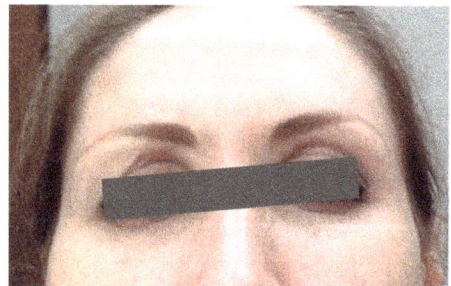

Figure II-2-6. Activation of additional agonist muscles: activation of the upper-lateral portion of the circular eye muscle during frowning after BoNT/A injection into the glabella region (adapted from Sharova A.A., Saromytskaya A.N., 2014)

During the initial examination, a detailed analysis of the patient's voluntary and involuntary facial expressions is needed to better understand the mechanisms of such muscle interactions. Expression tests are also required to detect latent hyperactivity of certain muscle areas and dynamic asymmetry before developing a BoNT/A injection regimen.

2.2.1. Activation of antagonist muscles

Clinical experience with BoNT/A for aesthetic indications shows that isolated correction of the frontalis muscle should never be attempted. Considering the patient's wishes, we can block the contractility of the interbrow depressor muscles without eliminating the activity of the frontalis muscle, but the reverse can never be achieved. By suppressing the activity of the frontalis muscle — the only levator of the upper third of the face — after the second or third BoNT/A injection, we will inevitably encounter increased activity and tone of the procerus and corrugator. This situation is clearly described by Kang S.M. et al. (2011), and their findings depicted in **Fig. II-2-7** show

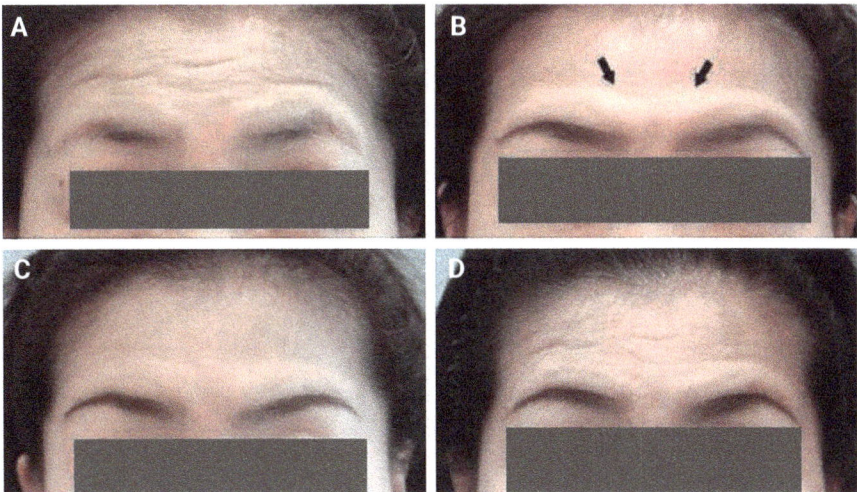

Figure II-2-7. (A) Patient with maximal forehead tension before treatment, (B) one week, (C) four weeks, and (D) 16 weeks after BoNT/A injections into the frontalis muscle (adapted from Kang S.M. et al., 2011)

that, in the absence of counteracting force after isolated correction of the frontalis muscle, the depressor muscles of the glabellar complex increase their activity and tone.

2.2.2. Activation of additional muscles

Another undesirable consequence of long-term BoNT/A use for aesthetic indications is activating additional muscle groups that do not have antagonistic relationships with the injected muscles. This usually occurs when the patient has hyperkinetic and/or hypertonic muscle activity (de Maio M., 2008). As the mimic "pattern" of emotional experience in such patients is overexpressed, the specialist's task is to gradually transform the type of mimic response into a normal kinetic one.

However, in some cases, during long-term botulinum therapy, the tone/activity of additional previously inactive muscles increases. In this way, the limitation of habitual mimic expression is compensated. In these individuals, owing to long-term isolated correction of the muscles of the upper third of the face, the activity of the depressors in the lower third of the face and their involvement in mimic reactions are frequently increased. Problems in the realization of a sincere smile (Duchenne smile*) against the background of prolonged relaxation of the lateral portion of the circular eye muscle lead to the formation of a bunny line against the background of activation of the nasal muscle or wrinkles at the inner corner of the eye due to the tension of the medial portion of the circular eye muscle (**Fig. II-2-8**).

In the lower third of the face, activation of the platysma often occurs (**Fig. II-2-9**) against the background of isolated correction of the muscle that lowers mouth corners (we consider these muscles as agonists in facial oval correction). To prevent undesirable phenomena caused by the activation of additional muscles, small doses of BoNT/A should be prophylactically injected into them to maintain

---

*Duchenne smile is named after 19th-century anatomist Guillaume Duchenne, who studied facial expressions. It is a type of smile involving specifically coded facial muscle expressions and is hypothesized to represent authentic positive displays of emotion. This kind of smile reaches your eyes and lights up your entire face.

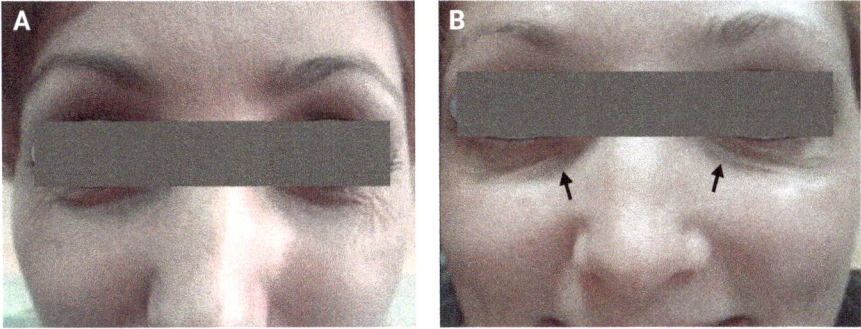

Figure II-2-8. Redistribution of muscle activity after BoNT/A injections in the area of "crow's feet": appearance of compensatory wrinkles in the medial corner of the eye (adapted from Sharova A.A., Saromytskaya A.N., 2014)

the balance of intermuscular relationships, but at a different level.

2.2.3. Activation of individual portions within a single muscle

When introducing BoNT/A into muscles in which individual portions have different contraction vectors, we often aim to weaken the activity of those muscle parts involved in the undesirable mimic activity.

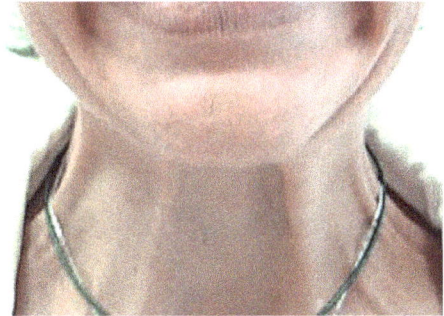

Figure II-2-9. Increase in platysma tone during isolated correction of muscles lowering the mouth corners (adapted from Sharova A.A., Saromytskaya A.N., 2014)

This effect is realized when working with the frontalis muscle, circular muscles of the eyes and mouth, levators of the upper lip and wing of the nose, as well as platysma. Similarly, the temporal muscles can be treated with BoNT/A, based on the assumption that the intact portion of the muscle takes on an "additional load" and its activity increases. We often get undesirable aesthetic effects in such a redistribution of muscle activity.

For example, activation of the inferior, levator, portion of the frontalis muscle was observed by Kang S.M. et al. (2011), who published photographs of one of their patients to show a noticeable crease above the eyebrow that appeared one week after BoNT/A injection into the superior portion of the frontalis muscle and spontaneously smoothed out after three weeks (see **Fig. II-2-2**). In our opinion, compensatory wrinkles over the lateral portions of the eyebrows may be related to overactivation of the lateral portion of the frontalis muscle after relaxation of its medial portion (where BoNT/A injection points were concentrated), especially in patients with high foreheads.

In patients with hyperactivity of the lower lateral portion of the circular eye muscle, especially in case of insignificant excess skin in the lower eyelid, "rigid" correction of the lateral portion of the circular eye muscle by introducing BoNT/A in three classical points leads to the redistribution of muscle activity and appearance of compensatory "incoming" wrinkles at the medial corner of the eye. In this situation, the ideal solution is to inject BoNT/A into the periorbital area using the superficial microinjection technique.

In practice, it is not uncommon to encounter increased tone of previously intact platysma bundles when BoNT/A is injected into initially visible overactive bundles (see **Fig. II-2-8**). Therefore, BoNT/A injections into the platysma are not as simple a clinical task as they may seem at first glance and may lead to the side effects associated with BoNT/A diffusion into deep muscles.

2.3. Changes in facial expression patterns

Facial expression patterns are characteristic wrinkle patterns associated with certain types of facial expression responses, degree of emotional expression, and features of facial muscles (Liang Y. et al., 2018).

It has been established that changes in facial expression patterns can occur under repeated BoNT/A administration (Nestor M.S. et al., 2020). Positive dynamics are associated with gradual weaning from the pathological habits of frowning, squinting, etc. Negative dynamics can be due to the activation of additional agonist muscles and, less often, antagonists, as discussed above. With repeated chemodenervation of the muscles of the interbrow region, there may be increased expression of the nasal muscles and the muscle that lifts the upper lip. In the lower third of the face, isolated denervation of the muscles lowering the mouth corners may be accompanied by an increased tone of the chin muscle and concomitant tonization of the platysma thrusts, which seem to continue the vector of contraction of the muscles lowering the mouth corners. In all these cases, we often observe the formation of new wrinkles or aggravation of the existing ones.

2.4. Changes in the emotional response

Above, we have discussed the potential positive effects on the patients' emotional background of BoNT/A injections into the muscles of the interbrow region, which are responsible for expressing negative emotions (Costa A.C.F. et al., 2022). However, we need to consider the possibility of the reverse situation — attenuating mimic expression and, therefore, the experience of positive emotions. By chemically denervating a single muscle, we inadvertently disrupt the well-coordinated habitual pattern of muscle contractions during mimic expression of feelings practiced for years. We have already mentioned the Duchenne smile, the realization of which involves not only the circular muscles of the mouth and the large and small zygomatic muscles but also the circular orbital muscle. It is the latter element that distinguishes a sincere smile associated with the experience of joy from a formal smile. Restricting the participation of the circular muscle of the eye in the expression of joyful emotions can theoretically, according to the feedback mechanism, weaken their experience. Such a situation is likely to occur when relatively large BoNT/A doses are administered, resulting in restricted mobility of the muscles of the upper third of the face.

Indeed, after a quite successful correction of the lower third of the face, associated with switching off (or weakening the activity of) the depressor muscles, some patients complain of an uncomfortable state associated with the expression of positive emotions. This adverse outcome occurs because some levator muscles in the middle third of the face begin to work more actively. As a result, the upper gum is exposed, and the upper lip is tucked in when smiling, which causes patients to experience certain discomfort. It is not uncommon to hear complaints of an "unnatural smile." Violation of the smile function is usually noticed by other people and their comments are perceived as extremely painful, negatively affecting the patient's quality of life. Moreover, due to the compensatory activation of some muscles, such as the upper lip, the neural pathways reflecting the conduction of negative emotions can theoretically be activated.

Résumé

Ample clinical experience in aesthetic botulinum therapy and an increasingly deep understanding of the mechanisms of BoNT/A action help physicians competently develop protocols for correcting expression lines and pharmacological facelifts. Accordingly, the preventive aspects of botulinum therapy are now receiving much greater attention.

Successful botulinum therapy implementation requires active interdisciplinary interaction among practitioners — skincare specialists, cosmetic dermatologists, neurologists, vertebrologists, and dentists. This is a significant incentive for continuous professional development because different specialists should speak the same "language."

Another emerging trend in this domain is the individualization of injection regimens to increase patient satisfaction and offset the negative aspects of long-term BoNT/A use. Orientation to standardized injection regimens and BoNT/A doses suggested by consensus of leading experts is an integral part of successful work. However, the recommended dose may be high or low for a particular individual. Neglecting the patient's characteristics may result in hypo- or hypercorrection of muscle activity. In the first case, this will lead to disappointment in the method or professionalism of the physician. Hypercorrection, especially if repeated many times, can lead to the formation and consolidation of unnatural facial expressions, resulting in negative changes in the emotion expression patterns.

Considering the reciprocal relationships of various mimic muscles, conscious management of their tone and activity makes it possible to not just smooth wrinkles but also harmonize and increase the aesthetic attractiveness of the human face both at rest and in facial expressions. It is often much more important to preserve a person's inherent charisma than to strive for radical wrinkle elimination. We hope that the generalizations and observations in this book section will prompt specialists to be more thoughtful and competent in their approach to botulinum therapy regimens.

Part III

Botulinum toxin and skin health

The growing body of scientific evidence on the effects of BoNT on the human body drives the expansion of medical indications for botulinum therapy. It has been established that this protein molecule can not only interrupt the transmission of nerve impulses in ACh-assisted synapses but may also influence other subtle mechanisms of intercellular interaction.

Thus far, research has demonstrated that BoNT inhibits the release of the neurogenic inflammatory mediators — substance P (SP) and calcitonin gene-related peptide (CGRP) — which allows its use in the treatment of various pain syndromes in neurology (Welch M.J. et al., 2000; Durham P.L., 2004).

BoNT blocks mast cells and prevents rosacea-like inflammation (Choi J.E. et al., 2019).

It also modulates wound healing processes not only through anti-inflammatory action, but also by influencing fibroblast activity and stimulating angiogenesis (Durham P.L., Cady R., 2004; Bansal C. et al., 2006).

The ability of BoNT to affect exocrine glands is widely used for treating hyperhidrosis (Henning M.A.S. et al., 2022). The same property allows BoNT/A preparations to be considered as a possible means for pathogenetic treatment of several dermatologic diseases — dyshidrotic eczema, multiple eccrine hydrocystoma, Frey syndrome (Laskawi R. et al., 1998; Laccourreye O. et al., 1999), Darier's disease, inverse psoriasis, aquagenic palm, and plantar keratoderma (Diba V.C. et al., 2005), familial benign vesicles (Hailey–Hailey disease), and some other conditions (Bansal C. et al., 2006; Messikh R. et al., 2009). Treating most of these conditions and diseases is beyond the responsibility and competence of an aesthetician. However, conditions that may be encountered in practice will be discussed in this part of the book (Hanna E., Pon K., 2020).

Prospective areas of research on the use of BoNT/A in cosmetic dermatology and aesthetic medicine

In dermatology (skin conditions and diseases to be treated):
- Raynaud's syndrome
- Dyshidrotic eczema
- Atopic dermatitis
- Psoriasis
- Itching
- Vasomotor disorders
- Scars
- Seborrhea
- Rosacea
- Acne
- Androgenetic alopecia
- Diffuse alopecia

In aesthetic medicine (treatment aims):
- Breast lifting
- Buttock lifting
- Leg curvature modification (change in the calf muscle shape)
- Post-acne treatment

Chapter 1
Rosacea

Rosacea is a chronic inflammatory disease of the facial skin characterized by the development of hyperemia (initially transient, then persistent), telangiectasias, papules and pustules, and, in later stages, tissue overgrowth and possible eye involvement (ophthalmic rosacea). This condition affects about 5% of adults worldwide, mainly those aged 45–60. While it was previously thought to be a disease of people of the "Celtic" type, modern data show that rosacea occurs in people of all phototypes. Nonetheless, it is much more noticeable in light-skinned people, who, therefore, tend to seek help in the early stages of the disease, while people with dark skin often come to physicians already exhibiting signs of progression (Buddenkotte J., Steinhoff M., 2018).

Rosacea can significantly impact the quality of life, with patients frequently reporting low self-esteem and decreased frequency of social interactions. Unfortunately, this dermatosis is untreatable, but it can (and should) be controlled so that the condition does not progress. Botulinum therapy may be one method of control.

1.1. Pathogenetic targets for BoNT

The skin of patients with rosacea is characterized by dysregulation of inflammatory (perivascular or perifollicular infiltrate), vascular (dilatation), lymphatic (dilatation), glandular (hyperplasia), and fibrotic processes.

Triggers (heat, ultraviolet/UV light, food, stress, irritants, infections, etc.) lead to the release of a whole group of mediators from keratinocytes, nerve, endothelial and mast cells, fibroblasts, and immune system cells (macrophages, Th1 and Th17 lymphocytes). These cells have specific receptors on their surface through which the action of the triggers is realized. In the case of rosacea, the receptors of the groups discussed below act as "intermediaries" between the trigger and the cell.

Toll-like receptors (TLRs) recognize microbial components, chemical and physical stimuli, and UV-induced apoptotic cells. TLR activation triggers pathogen-directed signaling cascades, including the secretion of antimicrobial peptides such as cathelicidin and the production of pro-inflammatory cytokines and chemokines (Meylan E. et al., 2006). Patients with rosacea have high levels of TLR-2 receptors, which begin to respond not only to microorganisms but also to many other triggering factors (heat, UV radiation, cold, alcohol). In this case, there is an increased expression of cathelicidin and kallikrein-5 (KLK-5), whereby the latter is cleaved by serine proteases to form the active peptide form of cathelicidin — LL-37 (Yamasaki K. et al., 2007). LL-37 stimulates leukocyte chemotaxis, angiogenesis, and capillary dilation, as well as activates MMPs that destroy the extracellular matrix (Yamasaki K. et al., 2007).

Transient receptor potential (TRP) channels are involved in response to heat, capsaicin, and other similar stimuli. Patients with erythematous-telangiectatic rosacea have an increased density of sensory neurons on which these receptors are located. In addition, transient receptor potential vanilloid subtype TRPV1, TRPV4, and TRPA1 receptors are situated on keratinocytes, endothelium, and mast cells (Sulk M. et al., 2012). TRP activation leads to the release of vasoactive neuropeptides such as SP, CGRP, vasoactive intestinal peptide, and pituitary adenylate cyclase-activating polypeptide. An increase in the levels of all these substances has been reported in rosacea (Rainer B.M. et al., 2017). SP is involved in the local regulation of blood flow and causes degranulation of mast cells, which leads to an increase in the level of pro-inflammatory cytokines (e.g., interleukins IL-1, IL-3, and IL-8), some chemokines, tumor necrosis factor-alpha (TNFα), and vascular endothelial growth factor (VEGF). All this confirms the presence of neurogenic inflammation in the pathogenesis of rosacea (Buddenkotte J., Steinhoff M., 2018).

In addition, the microbiome has also been implicated in the pathogenesis of rosacea with a long-known increase in the number of *Demodex* mites, but not only them. However, it is still unclear whether changes in the normal microbiome composition are a cause or a consequence of rosacea (Rainer B.M. et al., 2020).

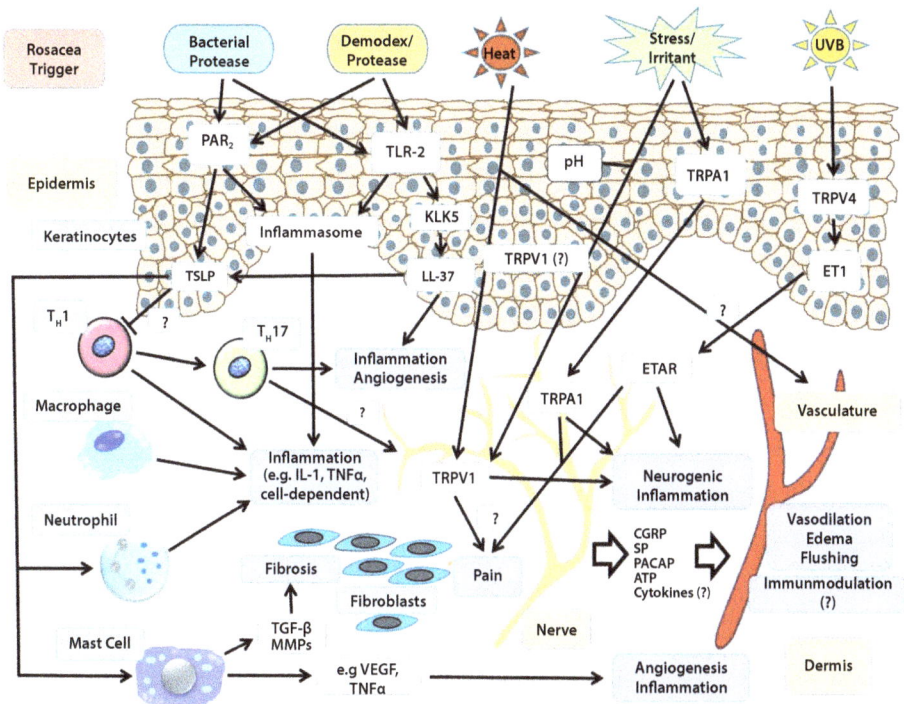

Figure III-1-1. Pathogenesis of rosacea (adapted from Buddenkotte J., Steinhoff M., 2018)

Rosacea triggers lead to the activation of downstream effectors (white boxes) in various cell types (gray boxes) probably by activating a few specific receptors and channels (white boxes), which in cooperation promote processes of (neurogenic) inflammation, including edema and vasodilation, fibrosis, pain, and angiogenesis (lilac boxes). For instance, epidermal and probably immune cell-expressed proteinase-activated receptor-2 (PAR2) and Toll-like receptor-2 (TLR-2) are activated by rosacea-associated bacterial and Demodex-derived proteases, leading to the induction of the inflammasome and subsequent release of pro-inflammatory agents such as tumor necrosis factor alpha (TNFα) and interleukin-1 (IL-1) as well as enhanced expression of the innate immune peptide LL-37. ATP — adenosine triphosphate; CGRP — calcitonin gene-related peptide; ET1 — endothelin-1; ETAR — endothelin A receptor; KLK-5 — kallikrein-5; LL-37 — cathelicidin; MMP — matrix metalloproteinase; NALP3 — NACHT, LRR, and PYD domain-containing protein 3; PACAP — pituitary adenylate cyclase-activating peptide; SP — substance P; TGF-β — transforming growth factor beta; TRP — transient receptor potential; TSLP — thymic stromal lymphopoietin; VEGF — vascular endothelial growth factor.

The pathogenesis of rosacea is summarized in **Fig. III-1-1** (Buddenkotte J., Steinhoff M., 2018). Rosacea may also be caused by impaired antioxidant defense. Studies have shown that rosacea patients have a genetically determined deficiency of the antioxidant defense system, namely a defective polymorphism of the enzyme involved in the formation of one of the key antioxidants — glutathione-S-transferase (Woo Y.R. et al., 2016). Under the action of reactive oxygen species (ROS), there is pronounced damage to the proteins and lipids of the epidermis, leading to the release of pro-inflammatory agents and triggering pathological reactions that involve keratinocytes, fibroblasts, and vascular endothelium of the skin. This cascade ultimately causes further aggravation of the aforementioned reactions.

One of the essential links in the disease pathogenesis is angioneurosis, which is a predominant lesion of facial vessels and is a manifestation of vegetovascular dystonia (Steinhoff M. et al., 2016). Vegetative dysfunctions contribute to the disruption of hemostasis and adaptation of the organism to various environmental influences, which leads to an increase in the permeability of the vascular wall, changes in the skin structure, and a decrease in the barrier function of the epidermis, thereby creating conditions for the development of inflammation in the skin.

Many clinical symptoms of rosacea occur via this mechanism. Due to the disruption of the connective tissue framework of the dermis, vessels dilate, and blood stagnates in them. Against the background of blood stasis, changes in the endothelium occur over time, and various inflammatory mediators begin to enter the perivascular space through the affected vascular wall, causing the formation of papules and pustules. Slow redistribution of blood flow and venous stasis in the outflow of facial angular veins (*vena facial sive angularis*) causes the most frequent topography of clinical manifestations of rosacea. The conjunctiva is also included in the area of facial vein outflow, which explains the frequent involvement of the eyes in this disease.

Thus, several rosacea subtypes can be diagnosed:

- **Erythematotelangiectatic** type — characterized by redness and persistent erythema in the central part of the face. Telangiectasias are common but are not mandatory for the diagnosis.
- **Papulopustular** type — manifests as papules, pustules, and erythema in the central area of the face.
- **Phymatous** type — distinguished by the thickening of the skin.
- **Ophthalmic (ocular) rosacea** — characterized by hyperemia of the eyelid conjunctiva, burning, and tingling.

1.2. Mechanism of BoNT action

The mechanism underlying the clinical effects of BoNT in rosacea still needs to be precisely defined. It is assumed that the inhibition of ACh release from peripheral nerve fibers, as well as inflammatory mediators SP and CGRP that modulate blood vessel dilatation, may play a role here.

Nerve endings of post- and preganglionic parasympathetic fibers release ACh, which affects organs by stimulating m- and n-cholinoreceptors. High-dose stimulation of m- and n-cholinoreceptors located in the ducts of sebaceous glands and vascular endothelium leads to the following changes:

- Inhibition of keratinocyte migration with subsequent follicular occlusion
- Increased secretory activity of sebaceous glands
- Release of SP — a neuropeptide involved in the regulation of secretory activity of holocrine glands and causing endothelium-dependent vasodilation
- Release of important inflammatory mediators (e.g., CGRP)
- Increased expression of certain types of receptor "mediators" such as TRPV1
- Release of nitric oxide (NO) — an endothelial relaxation factor that causes vasodilation

The anti-inflammatory effect of BoNT/A is due to the blockade of biological effects of SP, as well as thermoreceptors TRPV1 and CGRP. This reduces the severity of local subclinical inflammation manifested as erythema (Bansal C. et al., 2006). By blocking the ACh release, BoNT inhibits the release of NO by the endothelium.

Another possible mechanism described in a recent study concerns the effect of BoNT on mast cells, which are also involved in the pathogenesis of neurogenic inflammation in rosacea (Choi J.E. et al., 2019). Histamine released during their degranulation increases vascular wall permeability and contributes to itching. In their study, Choi J.E. et al. focused on the targeted effect of BoNT on human and mouse mast cells. For this purpose, the cells were treated with BoNT type A and B and a control solution, after which mast cell degranulation was induced by applying the compound 48/80*.

The obtained results indicated that preliminary exposure of cells to BoNT of both types significantly reduced the intensity of degranulation compared to the control group.

In addition, the scientists induced a rosacea-like condition in live mice using the active peptide of the antimicrobial protein cathelicidin LL-37, secreted in excess in rosacea. However, those previously receiving intradermal BoNT/A injections had significantly less erythema. They also had less pronounced mast cell degranulation and reduced mRNA expression of rosacea biomarkers such as KLK-5, MMP-9, and TRPV2, which are usually elevated in this disease (Choi J.E. et al., 2019).

These findings suggest that BoNT/A reduces rosacea-related skin inflammation by directly inhibiting mast cell degranulation. Choi J.E. and colleagues thus concluded that intradermal administration of the drug may help patients with refractory forms of rosacea. However, full-fledged clinical trials are needed to introduce the approach into widespread practice.

1.3. Clinical effects

As a part of a review published by an international team of scientists (Scala J. et al., 2019), studies on the use of BoNT in rosacea and facial hyperemia present in the International Database of Medical and Biological Research as of April 2017 were examined. The authors found 39 such articles, the first of which dated back to 2005, with 30 papers included in the final analysis. All investigations differed in the type and dosage of BoNT/A applied per cm^2 of the affected skin (1–6 IU), as well as the treatment frequency (one to three) and the interval between sessions (from two weeks to several months). Still, positive results were attained in all cases.

---

*Compound 48/80 triggers mast cell degranulation and promotes histamine release. It is widely used in animal and tissue models as a "selective" mast cell activator.

In only one of the studies included in the review, BoNT/A effects were evaluated according to the randomized controlled trial protocol (Odo M.E. et al., 2011). This investigation involved 60 menopausal women with menopausal hot flashes, 30 of whom were administered BoNT at fixed points, and the other 30 were given saline. At the control examination after 60 days, the BoNT-treated patients noted a significant reduction in the frequency and intensity of redness and sweating. While sweating returned after 180 days, it was less intense than before therapy.

As for rosacea specifically, a typical study with a single BoNT injection into the facial skin of 15 rosacea patients resulted in statistically significant reductions in erythema compared to baseline at 1, 2, and 3 months after treatment (Bloom B.S. et al., 2015).

Research on this topic is becoming more extensive, including double-blind, randomized trials, albeit with few participants. For example, Dayan S.H. et al. (2017) studied the efficacy of BoNT in nine patients with erythematotelangiectatic and papulopustular forms of rosacea. Four participants received BoNT/A injected into the cheek skin, while the remaining five received saline. Four weeks after the treatment, the experimental group showed a significant reduction in rosacea symptoms compared to the baseline and the control group.

Bharti J. et al. (2018) also reported on the effectiveness of BoNT intradermal injections. As a part of their study, microdroplets of BoNT/A solution were injected superficially (intradermally) into many points in small doses. The distance between injection points was 1 cm. The depth of injection, in this case, is of fundamental importance because in the cheek, mimic muscles bear a significant functional load. The introduction of the needle at a 75° angle to the skin surface and the release of a small part of the solution through the pores indicate an adequate injection depth. Two weeks after the procedure, the researchers recorded a significant reduction in erythema, edema, and redness outbreaks, as well as a decrease in rash and pore size. The effect persisted for 3–4 months (Bharti J. et al., 2018).

A clinical case from our practice involved a 28-year-old patient with the papulopustular form of rosacea with abscessation (**Fig. III-1-2A**) (Yutskovskaya Y.A. et al., 2016). Standard anti-inflammatory treatment

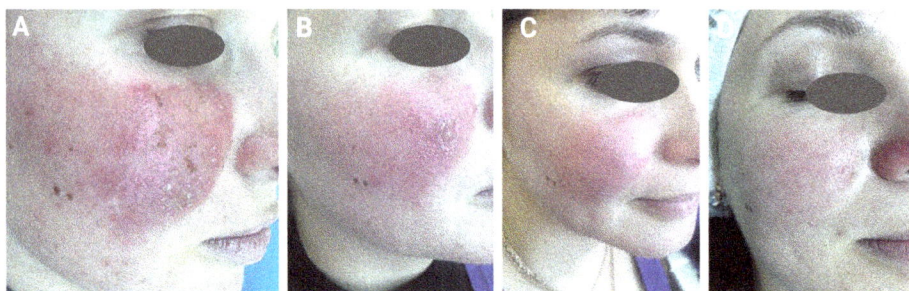

Figure III-1-2. Patient M., 28 years old. Ds: Rosacea (L71 according to International Classification of Diseases/ICD-10): (A) before initial treatment; (B) before the second treatment; (C) one month after the completion of botulinum therapy; (D) four months after the last treatment (adapted from Yutskovskaya J.A. et al., 2016)

Three BoNT/A microdroplet injection treatments in the cheek area were performed during remission. The interval between the first and the second procedure was 14 days, while that between the second and the third was 21 days. The preparation of abobotulinumtoxinA was injected in a 1:4 dilution with saline at a dose of 10 units per area; the total dose of the preparation for each procedure was 20 units.

aimed at inflammation control was performed in the first stage. The protocol involved intravenous injections of sodium thiosulfate five times every other day, along with metronidazole systemically (0.25 g three times a day for 14 days) and cryo-massage (10 procedures every other day). Further, three BoNT/A microdroplet injection treatments in the cheek area were carried out in the remission period. After the first treatment, a decrease in the number of acneiform rashes and a reduction in telangiectasias were noted (**Fig. III-1-2B**). Temporary erythema observed after the procedure lasted no more than an hour. After the course completion, the patient reported decreased flushes and improved skin texture and redness. The patient also experienced a decrease in wrinkles and pigment spots (**Fig. III-1-2C, D**).

Résumé

Although there have been no large-scale studies of the effect of BoNT on rosacea-affected skin, there are numerous reports in the medical press about its positive impact on the course of this very common chronic dermatosis (Zhang H. et al., 2021). Over the years, extensive clinical material on botulinum therapy for rosacea has been accumulated, confirming that this method is effective (He G. et al., 2024; Takahashi K.H. et al., 2024).

The currently known mechanisms of action suggest that BoNT has positive effects — after all, it affects one of the critical links in the pathogenesis of the disease. Therefore, botulinum injections may well be considered an element of the complex therapy for rosacea, but additional research is needed to develop standard protocols.

The *Rosacea and Couperosis in Cosmetic Dermatology & Skincare Practice* book provides more detailed information on rosacea.

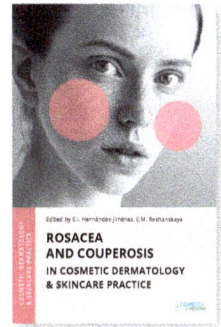

Chapter 2
Skin healing and scarring

Scar prevention and treatment are among the critical problems in aesthetic medicine. There is no single solution, and a combination of methods, selected individually, will be much more effective than monotherapy. Botulinum toxin has found a place in this therapeutic and preventive complex.

2.1. Normal and pathological scarring

To understand how BoNT intervenes in the scarring stage, let's trace the stages of skin repair from the beginning.

2.1.1. Stages of wound healing

Full-thickness wound healing is a dynamic and sequential process consisting of four stages — hemostasis, inflammation, proliferation, and remodeling. The entire cycle lasts about a year and culminates in mature scar formation (**Table III-2-1**).

Regardless of their localization, scars are dense lesions mainly composed of fibrous tissue. The epidermis covering the scar is depleted, the *stratum corneum* is altered, and its barrier properties are weakened.

A scar always occurs where the basal membrane is damaged, either linearly (in the case of a surgical incision or severe stretching — striae) or over a large area (after a burn). That is, scarring itself can be considered a normal phenomenon. If the scar is not very noticeable, does not limit movement, and does not change over time, it is regarded as a variant of the norm. However, not all scars behave predictably; some represent a pronounced aesthetic defect and create health problems.

Table III-2-1. Postoperative scarring

STAGE	MORPHOLOGY	CLINICAL PICTURE
Epithelization of the skin wound (1–10 days after surgery)	• Development and completion of postoperative inflammation • Formation of granulation tissue in the wound area • Epithelialization of the wound provided that its edges are matched	• After the sutures are removed, the wound edges may separate under even slight force • There's no scar yet
Fragile scar formation (10–30 days)	Maturation of granulation tissue and active fibrogenesis with the formation of a fragile scar	• The scar is tender, easily stretchable and highly visible
Solid scar formation (30–90 days)	An increase in the number of fibers in scar tissue, oriented in accordance with the dominant stretching direction	• The scar becomes firm and less noticeable • Under unfavorable wound healing conditions, hypertrophy of scar tissue or its transformation into a keloid develops
Final scar remodeling (3–12 months)	• Slow scar remodeling with increased longitudinal orientation of fibers • Scar tissue contains minimal cellular elements and single vessels	• The cutaneous normotrophic scar gradually reaches its maximal strength and becomes even less visible • Under unfavorable conditions, a hypertrophic or keloid scar is formed

2.2.2. Pathologic scars

Skin scars are considered pathologic when there is an apparent excess of connective tissue overgrowth (hypertrophic scar), its stiffness, and adhesion to the underlying structures, or, conversely, its deficiency (atrophic scar). Pathological scars also include keloid scars — according to modern concepts, keloids belong to pseudotumor fibromatoses (Viera M.H. et al., 2010; Berman B. et al., 2017). In all the above cases, there are disorders at one or another stage of wound healing, and hereditary predisposition to the formation of pathologic scars is often traced.

In medical literature, hypertrophic and keloid scars are combined into one group because both types are characterized by excessive fibrous tissue formation. However, there are significant differences between these types of scars, including in the clinical picture, which allows for differential diagnosis.

The growth of a hypertrophic scar begins immediately after healing. It is characterized by the formation of "excess tissue" over an area equal to the wound surface, while the borders of the keloid always extend beyond the area of injury. With hypertrophic scar, subjective sensations are absent or are insignificant. Keloid formations cause subjective sensations (itching, pain, skin tightness, paresthesias, etc.). Change in color of hypertrophic scars from pink to whitish occurs in the same manner as in normotrophic scars, and these scars noticeably regress and flatten over time. A keloid scar has an elastic consistency and uneven, slightly wrinkled surface. It remains saturated in color, does not spontaneously regress, and tends to overgrow.

Keloid scars are more common in those aged 10–30 years, while hypertrophic scars can manifest at any age. Pathological skin scars are often formed against the background of certain diseases (chickenpox, acne, pyoderma, skin tuberculosis, etc.), after severe trauma, burns, and surgical interventions, including those performed for aesthetic reasons.

The risk of pathological postoperative scarring is increased in case of infection, incision lines not in line with Langer skin tension lines, and deep wound closure with epidermal sutures only. If the wound is oriented along the fibers of the subcutaneous muscles (often, it corresponds to the Langer skin tension lines), then its edges will stretch in width insignificantly and the healing process will culminate in the formation of a normotrophic or atrophic scar. When the wound is oriented across the fibers of the subcutaneous muscles, there is a constant stretching-compression of the forming connective tissue. This leads to hyperstimulation of fibroplasia processes and increases the risk of hypertrophic scar formation, especially in facial expression areas.

Risk factors include a chronic inflammatory process maintained by micro tears of newly formed myofibrils during contraction of the mimic muscles. If skin incisions are made along Langer lines during surgery, this reduces the risk of scarring. When performing traumatic injuries and surgical interventions aimed at skin neoplasm removal, it is necessary to ensure immobilization of the damaged area to reduce tension on the wound edges.

2.2. Mechanism of action

As noted above, severe stretching of the wound edges inhibits its healing and can trigger processes leading to pathologic scar formation. Immobilization of the wound focus is typically carried out with the help of special incisions by applying different-level sutures but, in many cases, this is not enough. Numerous attempts to use pharmacological agents to correct wound convergence have also failed. Only after introducing BoNT/A preparations — long-acting local myorelaxants — into the practice of aesthetic medicine did the question of the possible use of botulinum therapy as a pathogenetic method of prevention and correction of pathologic scars come on the agenda.

BoNT/A injected into subcutaneous muscles (or even subcutaneously with subsequent diffusion into muscles) provides the effect of prolonged myorelaxation, due to which the skin is spread and is no longer stretched during facial expressions, i.e., long-term pharmacological immobilization (chemoimmobilization) of the skin takes place. Thus, BoNT/A injections at the stage of scar formation allow risk factors such as unfavorable scarring and excessive tissue tension to be excluded. Such prevention is especially relevant in case of surgical scar excision.

When BoNT/A is injected into the area of an already-formed atrophic scar, the skin surface is smoothed, and the scar becomes less prominent due to the relaxation of subcutaneous muscles. In the case of hypertrophic and keloid scars, BoNT/A injections can help reduce pain and improve the clinical picture. Scar deformities are especially noticeable in elderly patients when the thickness of skin and subcutaneous fay tissue is significantly reduced, and dense scar tissue is delineated from the surrounding skin against the background of muscle contractions. In this case, local myorelaxation can dramatically improve the skin's overall appearance (Goodman G.J., 2010).

The mechanism described above suggests an indirect effect of BoNT/A on fibroblasts through the weakening of external deforming forces to which these cells respond. However, research has shown that BoNT/A can act on fibroblasts directly. Specifically, Chen M. et al. (2016) found that BoNT/A not only suppresses the proliferation of fibroblasts isolated from hypertrophic scars but also stimulates their apoptosis. In the culture of cells isolated from the focus of scar contracture, under the action of BoNT/A, a pronounced inhibition of fibroblast proliferation and a decrease in the expression of actin and myosin in myofibroblasts — cells characteristic of hypertrophic scars — were observed by these authors. Likewise, Zhibo X. and Miaobo Z. (2008) noted fibroblasts' predominance at the cell cycle's resting stage in cultures isolated from hypertrophic scars treated with BoNT/A. At the same time, cells at different stages of mitosis prevailed in the untreated cell culture.

The mechanism of BoNT/A action on fibroblasts may involve the transforming growth factor TGF-β1. This factor plays a vital role in the formation of such scars — when its level increases, fibrosis begins. BoNT/A reduces the TGF-β1 expression in fibroblasts cultured *in vitro* (Sherris D.A., Gassner H.G., 2002; Gassner H.G. et al., 2006; Wilson A.M., 2006; Li Y.H. et al., 2021), and this process may be one of the molecular mechanisms of BoNT/A effect on hypertrophic scars. As for the fibroblasts of keloid scars, under the action of BoNT/A (injected into the scar area), there is a change in the expression of some genes responsible for proliferative processes — TGF-β1, VEGF, platelet-derived growth factor subunit A (PDGFA), MMP-1 — in the scar tissue (Xiaoxue W. et al., 2014).

Another aspect of the positive effect of botulinum therapy on scars relates to eliminating neurogenic symptoms: reduction of itching and skin tightness. This symptomatology is more characteristic of keloids but can also accompany emerging hypertrophic scars. In some cases, unpleasant sensations in the scar area lead to constant scratching, which aggravates the pathologic scarring process. In all cases, sensory disturbances cause suffering and reduce a patients' quality of life (Uyesugi B. et al., 2010). Yet, painful symptoms associated with keloid and hypertrophic scars are successfully managed with BoNT/A (Xiao Z. et al., 2009).

Although the mechanism of the analgesic action of BoNT/A is still not fully understood, we may assume that neurogenic inflammation is suppressed due to the blockade of transport proteins involved in the release of inflammatory neurotransmitters in the terminals of sensory nerves — SP, CGRP, and neurokinin (Bagues A. et al., 2024).

Initially, experiments exploring the direct effect of BoNT on cells were carried out on cell cultures. Over time, the focus shifted to the impact of BoNT/A on collagen deposition *in vivo*, as discussed below.

2.3. Histological studies

Xiao Z. and Qu G. (2012) conducted their studies on eight rabbits. Before administering BoNT/A, incisions were made deep to the cartilage on the ventral surface of both auricles. BoNT/A was injected into the scars on the right ear, whereas the left ear served as a control. The first BoNT/A injection was administered 28 days after the incision, and further two injections were performed at one-month intervals. Three months after the last injection, tissue samples were taken from the scar area for further analysis.

Even to the naked eye, the difference between BoNT/A-treated scars and the untreated controls was readily apparent (**Fig. III-2-1**). Direct

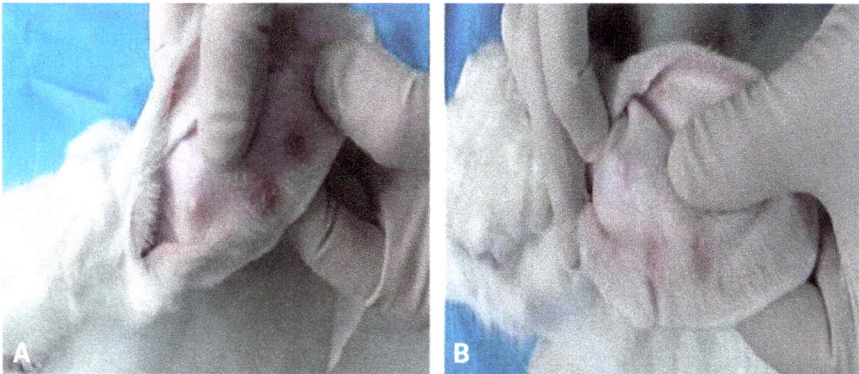

Figure III-2-1. Hypertrophic scar on the rabbit ear; observations were performed for six months after surgical skin injury: (A) control and (B) BoNT/A-treated scar (adapted from Xiao Z., Qu G., 2012)

Table III-2-2. Scar thickness with and without BoNT treatment (Xiao Z., Qu G., 2012)

SAMPLE NUMBER	1	2	3	4	5	6	7	8
Scar thickness without treatment (control), mm	1.92 ± 0.05	1.74 ± 0.03	1.57 ± 0.09	1.68 ± 0.02	1.37 ± 0.11	1.72 ± 0.8	1.64 ± 0.12	1.83 ± 0.09
Scar thickness after BoNT/A treatment, mm	0.90 ± 0.03	0.95 ± 0.18	1.16 ± 0.06	1.03 ± 0.11	1.08 ± 0.05	0.72 ± 0.09	0.69 ± 0.07	0.94 ± 0.02

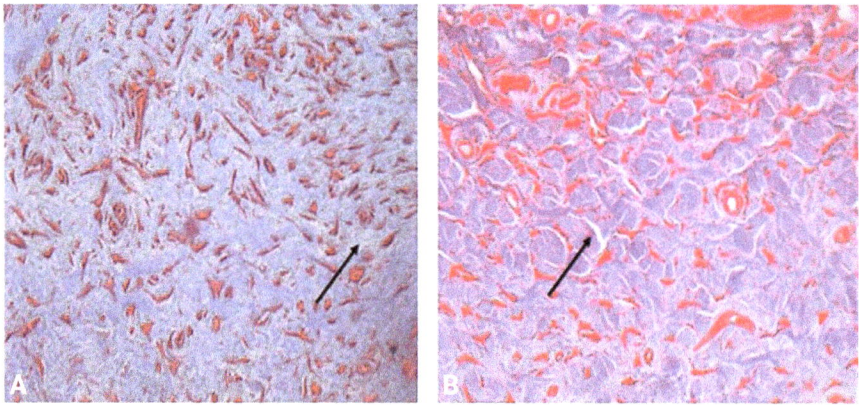

Figure III-2-2. Collagen fibers of hypertrophic scars (black arrow) in the control group are denser and more chaotically arranged than in the experimental group (Masson trichrome staining, 200×): (A) untreated scar (control) and (B) BoNT/A-treated scar (adapted from Xiao Z., Qu G., 2012)

measurements of scar thickness confirmed that the control scars were larger (**Table III-2-2**). Histological images show a difference in the structure of scar tissue — collagen fibers in the control group are thicker and more chaotically arranged than in BoNT/A-treated scars (**Fig. III-2-2**).

As scars localized on the auricular surface are practically unaffected by deforming forces, it can be assumed that, in this case, the effect is primarily related to other molecular and cellular mechanisms of BoNT/A's effect on fibroblasts.

2.4. Clinical observations

The scientific literature reports quite a few clinical observations on the effectiveness of botulinum therapy for scars. Still, according to most authors, BoNT injections are an auxiliary method of scar therapy and should be offered alongside steroid drugs and other treatment modalities (Sherris D.A., Gassner H.G., 2002; Bi M. et al., 2019; Sohrabi C., Goutos I., 2020).

2.4.1. Wound healing and scar prevention

Since 2000, several clinical studies have been conducted to investigate the effect of chemoimmobilization on the healing process of wounds caused by trauma or removal of facial neoplasms, as well as after plastic surgery, such as blepharoplasty (Yue S. et al., 2022) and laser skin resurfacing (Zhao P. et al., 2020). According to Wilson A.M. (2006), BoNT/A was injected into the mimic muscles 1–3 cm away from the wound edges to prevent scarring. After chemoimmobilization, wound healing with excellent aesthetic results was observed without adverse events. Wound localization perpendicular to the direction of muscle fibers suggests the most effective use of BoNT/A, especially in the frontal region. Chemodenervation of subcutaneous muscles before surgical intervention forms an aesthetically acceptable scar in 90% of cases. Several authors also noted that BoNT/A injections into the circular muscle of the mouth before surgical correction of congenital cleft lip provide a pronounced effect of wound tension reduction and cosmetic scar formation (Tollefson T.T. et al., 2006; Bartkowska P. et al., 2020).

Specialists of the Department of Otolaryngology at the Mayo Clinic (USA) have shown that injecting BoNT into the area of a forming scar on the face (caused by trauma, animal bite, biopsy, neoplasm excision) provides favorable conditions for healing, resulting in the formation of a normotrophic scar. The results of a prospective blind randomized clinical trial involving 31 patients conducted at the Mayo Clinic fully confirmed these findings (Gassner H.G. et al., 2006).

2.4.2. Scar revision

According to many experts, following the excision of pathologic scars, BoNT/A can be administered intradermally immediately after suturing or suture removal (Goodman G.J., 2010). However, even superficial injection of the drug does not prevent its diffusion into deeper tissue layers and subsequent relaxation of functionally important muscles. Therefore, such injections are not performed in the cheek area. At the same time, adequate correction of scars in the forehead, chin, and interbrow area contributes not only to the improvement of scar appearance but also to wrinkle smoothing in the injection areas.

BoNT/A injections can also be administered into the scar tissue for effective pain management (Carruthers A. et al., 2022). Indeed, some patients do not notice a clinically significant improvement in the appearance of the scar but report a reduction in pain.

Xiao Z. et al. (2009) observed 19 patients after BoNT/A injection into hypertrophic scar tissue. For six months, the clinical picture changed favorably (scars became soft, tissues became more mobile, and itching and erythema decreased), and all patients expressed high satisfaction with the therapy.

Concerning keloid scars, there is currently no consensus among experts as to whether botulinum therapy should be included in the treatment plan (Sohrabi C., Goutos I., 2020). Nonetheless, some encouraging clinical observations suggest that BoNT might be beneficial even in these cases.

For example, in the study conducted by Zhibo X. and Miaobo Z. (2009), 12 patients were injected with BoNT directly into the keloid scar tissue. The procedures were performed several times at three-month intervals. One year after the course completion, three patients had excellent results, five had good results, and four had satisfactory results. None of the observed clinical pictures returned to the initial level.

As a part of their investigation, Robinson A.J. et al. (2013) treated 12 patients with keloid scars on different body parts resistant to prior treatments. The patients were provided with a combination of intrafocal injections of triamcinolone acetonide and BoNT/A injections into the scar area. In all cases, therapy resulted in a pronounced scar regression — reduction in size, pallor, and texture softening, which was generally reflected in a significant decrease in the Vancouver scale score. Undesirable events were observed in four cases: scar formation in adjacent areas in two patients, steroid-induced atrophy of the skin in one patient, and skin ulceration in another patient who had previously received intense pulsed light (IPL) therapy. According to some authors, BoNT/A injections into the area of keloid scars also reduce adverse sensations such as pain, burning, and itching (Uyesugi B. et al., 2010).

However, several studies contrast these views. For instance, as a part of their research at the Ludwig Maximilian University (Munich, Germany), Gauglitz G.G. et al. (2012) didn't note any significant effect of botulinum monotherapy on the condition of keloid scars. Their findings also challenged the assumption that BoNT/A injected into the keloid scar area reduces the TGF-β1 expression and inhibits fibroblast proliferation.

Today, botulinum therapy is increasingly combined with energy-based physical treatments, fractional photothermolysis in particular. The effectiveness of such method combinations in the correction of age-related skin changes is well established (Carruthers J., Carruthers A., 1998, 2000; West T.B., Alster T.A., 1999; Yamauchi P.S. et al., 2004; Boughdadi N.S., Sadek E.Y., 2010; Zimbler M., Undavia S., 2012). According to the treatment protocols proposed by the authors of most publications, botulinum therapy precedes laser exposure, and the rationale for this course design is to optimize conditions for subsequent healing (Yao B. et al., 2023).

Résumé

The appropriateness of botulinum therapy in the treatment of pathologic scars remains a subject of research and debate. Analyzing the known data, we can come to the following conclusions:
1. The efficacy of BoNT/A injections into scar tissue at the formation stage to prevent pathological growth has been confirmed by several well-designed clinical studies (Goodman G.J., 2010; Liu A. et al., 2011; Al-Qattan M.M. et al., 2013; Ziade M. et al., 2013; Kim Y.S. et al., 2014; Yue S. et al., 2022).

2. Clinical practice shows that BoNT/A injections into the area of an already-formed hypertrophic scar contribute to its flattening, tissue softening, and visual improvement of the problem area (Xiao Z. et al., 2009). However, this conclusion is questioned due to the subjectivity of the methodology for assessing the state of the scar on the Vancouver scale (Freshwater M.F., 2013).
3. There is no consensus on the suitability of BoNT/A injections for keloid scars (Sohabi C., Guotos I., 2020). There are some publications describing positive clinical experiences (Zhibo X., Miaobo Z., 2009), but there are also reports refuting the efficacy of BoNT injections as a monotherapy for keloid scars (Gauglitz G.G. et al., 2012).
4. The maximal effect is achieved through combined treatment, in which botulinum therapy is one of the methods.

For more detailed information on scars, see the *Scars and Striae in Cosmetic Dermatology & Skincare Practice* book.

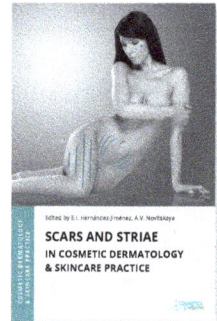

Edited by E.I. Hernández-Jiménez, A.V. Novitskaya

SCARS AND STRIAE
IN COSMETIC DERMATOLOGY
& SKINCARE PRACTICE

Chapter 3
Pigmentation

Until recently, there was no clinical explanation for the fact that **multiple intradermal BoNT injections lighten and even out the skin tone** whereas no such effect is observed with intramuscular injections! Most scientists assumed that BoNT is able to affect skin melanocytes and tyrosinase activity (Friedland S., Burde R.M., 1996; Carruthers J., Carruthers A., 2004; Yamauchi P.S. et al., 2004), but convincing evidence and understanding of how this occurs has been lacking. Consequently, there was no basis for developing practice guidelines and protocols.

The work of Korean scientists Jung J.A. et al. (2019), published in the Journal of Plastic and Reconstructive Surgery, allowed us to make significant progress in understanding the molecular and cellular mechanisms of BoNT's action on skin cells and to reach practical conclusions regarding the possibility of using BoNT to treat pigmentation.

3.1. Effect of BoNT on melanogenesis

3.1.1. Study design

Jung J.A. et al.'s (2019) study was conducted in two phases: *in vitro* — on mixed culture containing human keratinocytes and melanocytes, and *in vivo* — on animal models (mice).

In the first step, the authors co-cultured epidermal melanocytes with human keratinocytes to mimic natural cell-to-cell interactions. Epidermal melanocytes are cells localized at the basal level of the epidermis, capable of producing melanin pigment and interacting with keratinocytes through melanocyte outgrowths — dendrites. Melanin "packed" in melanosomes is transferred to keratinocytes around the nucleus to protect it from UV radiation. After 24 hours, some of the cells in the mixed culture were treated with BoNT/A, while the other part served as a control and remained intact. Next, all cells were exposed to ultraviolet type B (UVB) radiation at different doses before being incubated again. Melanocyte proliferation, morphology and number of dendrites, tyrosinase activity, and melanin level content were further evaluated, and immunofluorescence analysis was performed to assess the ability of BoNT/A to penetrate cells.

In the *in vivo* part of the study, BoNT/A was injected into the skin on one side of each animal's back while the other remained intact (control). One week after the BoNT/A injection, the skin on both sides was exposed to UVB radiation. The degree of skin pigmentation, histologic changes, and the number of dihydroxyphenylalanine/DOPA-positive melanocytes (the presence of DOPA is a marker of active melanogenesis) were evaluated. The level of pro-inflammatory cytokines — basic fibroblast growth factor (bFGF), IL-1α, and PGE$_2$ — was also analyzed.

3.1.2. Results

A comprehensive quantitative and qualitative evaluation of the major skin cells involved in the process of melanogenesis revealed many interesting findings, as outlined below.

Impact on melanocyte proliferation and the number of their dendrites

In the BoNT/A-treated mixed cell culture, the number of melanocytes was slightly lower after UVB irradiation relative to the untreated control, but their outgrowth (average number of dendrites per cell) was markedly lower than in the control (**Fig. III-3-1**), making it difficult for melanosomes to transfer to keratinocytes.

BoNT/A uptake by melanocytes and keratinocytes

To assess the ability of BoNT/A to penetrate various cells, immunofluorescence analysis was performed using cultured human neuroblastoma SH-SY5Y cells as a positive control and human dermal

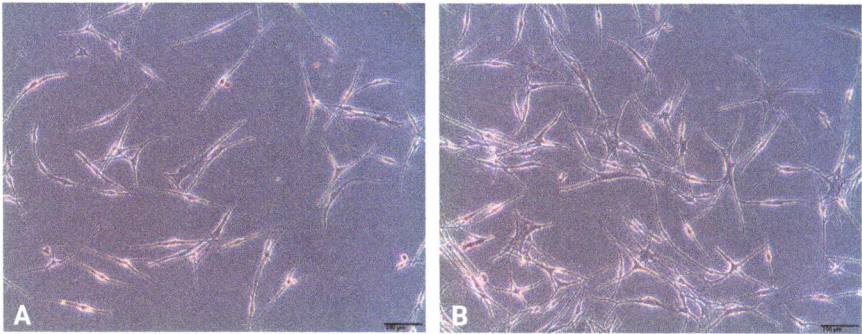

Figure III-3-1. Epidermal melanocyte outgrowth after UV irradiation. (A) Pre-cultivation with BoNT/A reduces the number of melanocyte outgrowths compared to (B) untreated control (adapted from Jung J.A. et al., 2019)

fibroblasts as a negative control. These cells were chosen because melanocytes, like neurons, are of ectodermal origin. Their connections with keratinocytes via dendrites are very similar to neuromuscular connections, the signal transmission between which is blocked by BoNT/A.

Significant amounts of BoNT/A were recorded in neuroblastoma cells, keratinocytes, and melanocytes, but no BoNT/A was found in dermal fibroblasts.

Impact on melanin content and tyrosinase activity in human epidermal melanocytes

In human epidermal melanocytes treated with BoNT/A, the melanin content averaged 94.0% (79.0–119.5%), significantly lower than that of the control (117.0%; 111.0–146.0%). However, tyrosinase activity in treated melanocytes was 107.0% (71.0–109.5%), while 94.0% (82.5–110.0%) was noted in controls, but these differences were not statistically significant.

Thus, treating cells with BoNT/A reduces their melanin content but does not affect tyrosinase activity.

Impact on UVB radiation-induced skin pigmentation in mice

In the *in vivo* experiments, the BoNT/A-injected side showed less intense pigmentation after UVB exposure than the control side, where BoNT/A was not injected (**Fig. III-3-2**).

Impact on the number of DOPA-positive melanocytes in mouse skin

On the dorsal side of the BoNT/A-treated mice, a decrease in the accumulation of melanin granules in the epidermis was observed after UVB irradiation compared with the control. The number of DOPA-positive melanocytes in the BoNT/A injection area was also significantly lower than on the control side (**Fig. III-3-3**).

As DOPA serves as a marker of active melanogenesis, a decrease in the number of DOPA-positive melanocytes indicates inhibition of melanin formation from tyrosine by tyrosinase and DOPA-oxidase enzymes.

Impact on melanin content and tyrosinase activity *in vivo*

The epidermis of BoNT/A-treated skin had a melanin content of 20.49 μg/mg (13.2–40.91 μg/mg), which was significantly lower than 31.13 μg/mg (25.91–81.31 μg/mg) measured on the control side. Tyrosinase activity was also considerably lower in the treated skin, indicating decreased melanin synthesis due to BoNT/A.

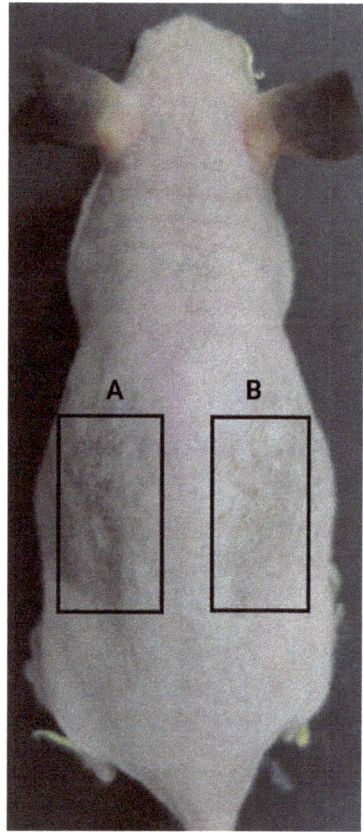

Figure III-3-2. Effect of BoNT/A on the degree of skin pigmentation in mice after UVB irradiation (Jung J.A. et al., 2019). Pre-administration of BoNT/A reduces the ability of skin to produce pigment under UVB exposure: (A) UVB alone (control); (B) BoNT/A + UVB (adapted from Jung J.A. et al., 2019)

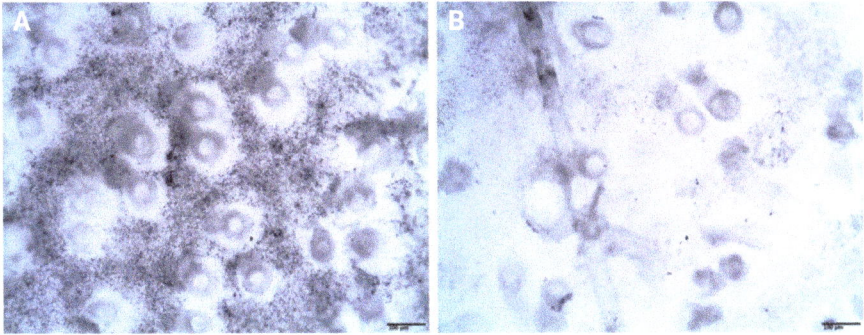

Figure III-3-3. Evaluation of the number of DOPA-positive melanocytes. BoNT/A pre-injection reduces the number of active DOPA-positive melanocytes in the epidermis: (A) UVB alone (control); (B) BoNT/A + UVB (adapted from Jung J.A. et al., 2019)

Impact on the concentration of mediators regulating inflammation

On the side of BoNT/A administration, there was a significant decrease in the levels of the pro-inflammatory cytokines — bFGF, IL-1α, and PGE_2 (**Fig. III-3-4**).

bFGF production occurs in normal tissue and is activated in chronic inflammatory reactions.

IL-1α is a potent inflammatory cytokine that activates the inflammatory processes in the body. Unregulated intracellular signal transduction involving IL-1α causes skin pathologies accompanied by severe acute or chronic inflammation.

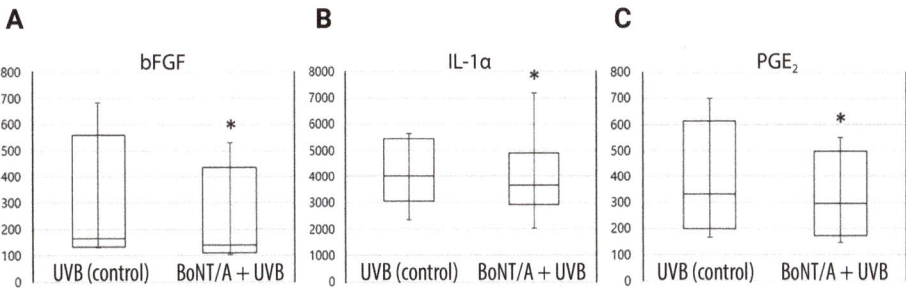

Figure III-3-4. Evaluation of inflammatory mediator levels in the skin of mice after UVB irradiation: ((A) bFGF, (B) IL-1α, and (C) PGE_2 (adapted from Jung J.A. et al., 2019)

PGE$_2$, in turn, is the most common prostaglandin (PG) secreted by keratinocytes after UV irradiation. It acts on melanocytes by stimulating tyrosinase activation.

It is known that any type of inflammation, including that induced by UV exposure, can lead to the development of post-inflammatory hyperpigmentation. Accordingly, reduction in the amount of pro-inflammatory cytokines under the influence of BoNT/A will also lessen the severity of pigmentation.

3.2. Is botulinum toxin a skin protector against UV-induced pigmentation?

As shown above, Jung J.A. et al.'s (2019) study has partially explained the skin pigmentation lightening commonly observed in clinical practice after multiple intradermal BoNT/A injections. They demonstrated that BoNT/A can penetrate not only neurons but also melanocytes and block the transfer of melanosomes from melanocyte dendrites to keratinocytes. Still, it is not precisely known how this blockade occurs and what is targeted by BoNT/A within the dendrite. However, since melanocytes and neurons have the same ectodermal origin, it is possible that mediator release from the nerve endings and melanosome exit from the dendrite proceed via similar mechanisms.

As for the decrease in the number of melanosomes and tyrosinase activity in melanocytes in the skin treated with BoNT/A before UV irradiation, it may be attributed to the reduced production of cytokines (including the pro-inflammatory ones) in keratinocytes. The fact is that when the skin is exposed to UV rays, keratinocytes are the first to sense it and, in response, produce signaling substances that trigger melanin synthesis in melanocytes. Keratinocyte sensitivity to UV radiation decreases after BoNT/A treatment, as does the release of signaling molecules, which prevents melanocytes from receiving the proper signal for activation.

The subtle molecular and cellular mechanisms underlying these processes have yet to be studied. Nonetheless, it has already been experimentally confirmed that, after BoNT/A treatment, the skin's ability to synthesize pigment is reduced (Erdil D. et al., 2023). On the one hand, these observations open the prospect of developing new protocols in aesthetic botulinum therapy. On the other hand, they indicate the necessity of mandatory use of sunscreen during the entire duration of BoNT/A action — as was shown in the studies mentioned above, during this time, the skin's ability to produce its photoprotective pigment decreases.

3.3. Topical botulinum toxin application for skin lightening: rationale and practical recommendations

If we consider botulinum therapy for age spot prevention and correction, **injecting BoNT/A has a disadvantage**: any injection is an injury that provokes an inflammatory response. Since inflammation activates melanogenesis, non-invasive topical application of BoNT/A is preferable.

The first and so far the only topical botulinum therapy technology of its kind has already appeared on the market (see Part V, section 1.2). One of its clinical effects is lightening pigmentation and evening the skin tone (**Fig. III-3-5**). This is particularly relevant for acne

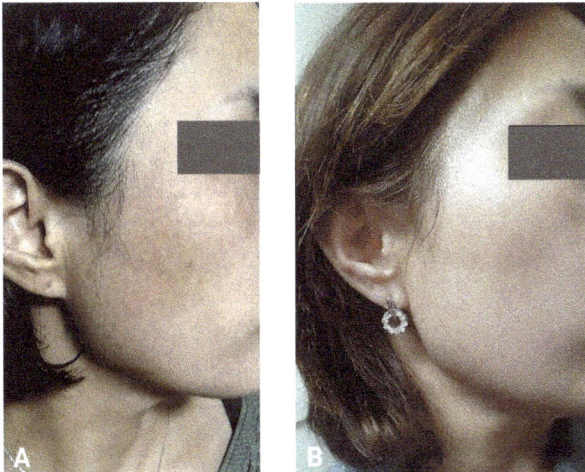

Figure III-3-5. Lightening of melasma: (A) initial skin condition; (B) after four months of daily application of cosmetic products with BoLCA — recently developed compound containing botulinum toxin light chain type A (Lee B.K., 2020)

and post-acne patients in whom pigmentation is of inflammatory origin (Lee B.K., 2019), as well as for those planning aesthetic procedures associated with inflammation, such as microdermabrasion, mesotherapy, fractional radiofrequency (RF) therapy, fractional photothermolysis. In all these cases, topical botulinum toxin is recommended during the rehabilitation phase to reduce inflammation and the associated risks of post-inflammatory pigmentation.

Another essential practical point has become apparent from extant research. During topical botulinum therapy, broad-spectrum (UVA/B) photoprotective agents are mandatory to reduce the UV load on the skin, and antioxidant supplements are advised to prevent oxidative stress and reduce inflammation. Such external assistance is essential for skin with a reduced intrinsic photoprotective capacity for pigment production (Lee B.K., 2020).

Résumé

Through direct and indirect mechanisms, BoNT/A can reduce pigmentation *in vitro* and *in vivo*.

The direct mechanism probably arises because melanocytes, like neurons, are of ectodermal origin, and their connections to keratinocytes via dendrites are very similar to neuromuscular connections, the signal transmission between which is blocked by BoNT/A.

An indirect mechanism is related to the identified anti-inflammatory effects of BoNT/A.

Further clinical studies are needed to develop qualitatively new methods to control UV-induced skin pigmentation using BoNT/A.

More information on pigmentation is available in our *Pigmentation in Cosmetic Dermatology & Skincare Practice* book.

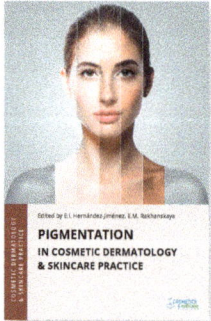

Edited by E.I. Hernández Jiménez, E.M. Nakhankaya

PIGMENTATION
IN COSMETIC DERMATOLOGY
& SKINCARE PRACTICE

Chapter 4
Oily skin

Oily skin associated with overactive sebaceous glands is one of the most common complaints for which patients seek help from aestheticians and dermatologists. Oily skin has a characteristic appearance — it is gleaming, its pores are enlarged, it may be prone to sizeable scaly flaking, and it acquires a "dirty" yellowish–grayish color in light phototypes. In addition to the aesthetic aspect, oily skin is prone to irritation and may develop acne, seborrheic dermatitis, or both.

Changes in the functioning of sebocytes — the cells that secrete sebum — are associated with dysregulation of the sebaceous glands when, for one reason or another, they receive more stimulating "signals." However, clinical observations and experimental studies have shown that BoNT can help control this condition.

How does it manage to do that?

4.1. Mechanism of action

The autonomic nervous system — neither sympathetic nor parasympathetic — is known to have a direct stimulatory effect on the sebaceous glands. At the same time, the nicotinic acetylcholine receptor α7 (nAchRα7) — a representative of the group of n-choline receptors, which is activated not only by nicotine but also by ACh — has been found on the membrane of sebocytes. The nAchRα7 receptors have been identified in sebocytes at different stages of development, but their number is higher on the membrane of the mature ones. Moreover, the number of these receptors in the sebocytes of normal skin is lower than in oily skin (Zouboulis C.C. et al., 2008).

In addition to expressing cholinergic receptors, sebocytes can produce and release ACh. ACh promotes sebocyte maturation and division, and in mature sebocytes it increases lipid synthesis via the extracellular signal-regulated kinase (ERK) signaling pathway*, leading to the inhibition of peroxisome proliferator-activated receptor gamma (PRAR-γ). Research has shown that sebocytes within the sebaceous gland can auto-stimulate with the help of the mediator they produce when exposed to acetylcholine (Kurzen H. et al., 2004; Li Z.J. et al., 2013).

BoNT can block the cholinergic auto-stimulation of sebocytes. Since oily skin has much more mature sebocytes than normal skin, intradermal BoNT injections reduce sebum production in oily skin and are hardly noticeable in normal skin.

It is also interesting to note that sebaceous glands are located between the hair follicles and the muscle that lifts the hair (*m. arrector pili*), which is stimulated by adrenaline and the sympathetic nervous system. This muscle is probably involved not only in evacuating sebum from the gland duct to the skin surface but also in regulating sebum production in the sebocytes (Song W.C. et al., 2007). There is also an assumption that BoNT affects *m. arrector pili* through local muscarinic receptors in the sebaceous gland (Rose A.E., Goldberg D.J., 2013).

Still, while the cellular targets inside the skin are known, the fine molecular details are missing. In the nerve cell, the molecular targets for BoNT are the proteins of the SNARE complex, and disruption in any one of these proteins makes it impossible for the ACh-loaded synaptic vesicle to dock with the presynaptic membrane and release the mediator into the synaptic cleft. What is the molecular target in the sebocyte or sebaceous gland-adjacent structures? We do not yet know — this remains to be studied.

4.2. Clinical effects

Shah A.R. (2008) was the first to propose intradermal microdose BoNT injections to treat oily skin and prevent enlarged pore formation.

---

*The ERK pathway plays an important role in integrating external signals from the presence of mitogens such as epidermal growth factor (EGF) into signaling events promoting cell growth and proliferation in many mammalian cell types. The ERK pathway is an information superhighway between the surface membrane and the nucleus, and it effectively links environmental signals to genomic responses. After activation, cytoplasmic ERK translocates to the nucleus, where ERK activates specific transcription factors to regulate gene transcription. — Wikipedia

The evidence supporting this method was acquired by providing one intradermal botulinum injection in the T-zone to 20 patients with oily skin and a history of enlarged pores, and the results were evaluated by clinical photography 30 days later. Although 17 of these patients reported improved skin condition and reduced oiliness, the author acknowledged limited generalizability of these findings due to the retrospective study design and the lack of objective analysis of sebum production.

Nevertheless, a new trend has been set, prompting research into BoNT use in skincare. Since then, many clinical papers have been published, relying on patients' subjective opinions and visual analyses and measurement data (Dayel S.B. et al., 2024). In all known articles on the subject, the efficacy and safety of intradermal microdose botulinum therapy in oily skin were demonstrated (Shuo L. et al., 2019; Rho N.K., Gil Y.C., 2021; Calvisi L. et al., 2022).

Thus, we can conclude that topical botulinum toxin has also shown promise in controlling sebum. Although regular and long-term use of cosmetic products containing it is needed to achieve meaningful results, it can be used between botulinum injection treatments to maintain clinical effects (Lee B.K., 2019, 2020).

Résumé

Studies on the use of BoNT to control sebum production are ongoing. The clinical effect and safety have been confirmed, and the cellular targets are known. However, the subtle molecular mechanisms remain to be uncovered to complete the picture and justify the feasibility of including botulinum therapy in the clinical guidelines for oily skin treatment.

Our *Oily Skin, Acne, And Post-Acne in Cosmetic Dermatology & Skincare Practice* book discusses oily skin and related disorders in more detail.

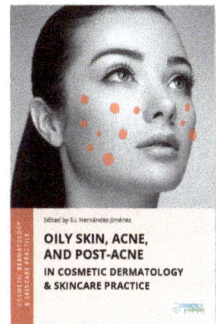

Edited by I.I. Hernández-Jiménez

OILY SKIN, ACNE, AND POST-ACNE
IN COSMETIC DERMATOLOGY & SKINCARE PRACTICE

Chapter 5
Hyperhidrosis

Hyperhidrosis is a functional disorder resulting in profuse sweating as a reaction to external stimuli or a consequence of disease. Hyperhidrosis affects about 3% of people in the general population, with 1.5 times greater prevalence in men than women (Callejas M.A. et al., 2010).

Depending on its cause, hyperhidrosis is divided into primary (essential) and secondary (developed against the background of other diseases), and by prevalence — into generalized and localized (**Table III-5-1**).

Primary hyperhidrosis is the most common sweating disorder, primarily affecting axillae, palms, and feet. In patients with primary hyperhidrosis, the number of sweat glands is increased, and their sensitivity and strength of response to everyday stimuli are also heightened. As a rule, primary hyperhidrosis initially manifests in childhood and dramatically intensifies during puberty. When making the "primary hyperhidrosis" diagnosis, it is necessary to exclude several diseases of neurological, endocrine, and somatic nature, as these are causes of secondary hyperhidrosis. Thus, the following criteria for the diagnosis of primary local hyperhidrosis should be considered (Hornberger J. et al., 2004):

1. Localized excessive sweating for at least six months
2. Absence of causes for secondary hyperhidrosis
3. At least two of the following characteristics:
   - Bilateral and relatively symmetric process
   - Debut at less than 25 years of age
   - Family history of primary localized hyperhidrosis
   - Cessation of localized sweating during sleep
   - Frequency of manifestations — at least one episode per week
   - Disruption of daily activities

Table III-5-1. Causes of generalized and localized forms of hyperhidrosis (Glaser A., Naumann M., 2009)

GENERALIZED HYPERHIDROSIS	LOCALIZED HYPERHIDROSIS
• High body temperature / fever • Infections • Malignant diseases, tumors • Thyrotoxicosis • Pheochromocytoma • Diabetes mellitus • Hypoglycemia • Hypopituitarism • Endocarditis • Gout • Drugs: antimuscarinic anticholinergic agents, carbonic anhydrase inhibitors, and tricyclic antidepressants • Menopause • Anxiety • Withdrawal syndrome*	• Primary localized hyperhidrosis • Localized unilateral hyperhidrosis • Tumors of intrathoracic localization • Rheumatoid arthritis • Spinal cord diseases or injuries • Stroke • Syringomyelia • Ross syndrome** • Atrioventricular fistula • Frey syndrome*** • Cold hyperhidrosis • Eccrine nevus • Social phobia (anxiety disorder)

*Withdrawal syndrome, also known as discontinuation syndrome, occurs when individuals discontinue or reduce their use of a substance to which they have developed physiological dependence.

**Ross syndrome is a rare peripheral autonomic nervous system disorder characterized by three features: tonic (Adie) pupil(s), reduced or loss of deep tendon reflexes (hyporeflexia or areflexia), and segmental anhidrosis.

***Frey syndrome (gustatory sweating) manifests as unilateral perspiration and flushing of the facial skin during meals.

Gustatory sweating (Frey syndrome) is a special type of hyperhidrosis. Its main symptom is the appearance of profuse sweating in the cheek and parotid region during salivation when eating or waiting for a meal. This disorder may occur as a complication of surgical treatment of parotid salivary gland diseases or because of facial trauma (Hartl D.M. et al., 2008).

Various quantitative and qualitative methods, such as the ninhydrin test and sudomotor axon reflex tests, are used to assess sweating intensity. Still, in clinical practice, the **iodine–starch test (Minor test)** is most frequently conducted (**Fig. III-5-1**).

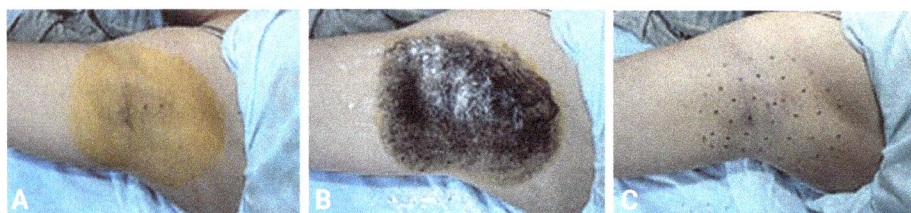

Figure III-5-1. Minor test in axillary hyperhidrosis: (A) the zone of increased sweating is treated with Lugol's solution; (B) after application of potato starch in the zone of sweating, purple–black staining appears; (C) BoNT injection points (adapted from Artemenko A.R., 2011)

Treatment for excessive sweating depends on the form of hyperhidrosis (Vorkamp T. et al., 2010). In secondary hyperhidrosis, the priority is given to controlling the underlying disease. As a conservative treatment, topical agents containing solutions of aluminum salts, zirconium, glutaric aldehyde, tannic acid, etc., are used, as well as oral drugs of systemic action, such as cholinolytics, β-adrenoblocators, tranquilizers, calcium channel blockers, and agonists of α2-adrenoreceptors. However, the effectiveness of such drugs is limited, and their use often leads to undesirable adverse reactions. Among the physical methods for treating hyperhidrosis, iontophoresis appears to be most beneficial.

Nonetheless, surgical intervention and intradermal BoNT/A injections remain the most effective hyperhidrosis treatment methods (McConaghy J.R., Fosselman D., 2018). Regarding the surgical therapies for localized hyperhidrosis, the best results are achieved with transthoracic endoscopic sympathectomy. The procedure lasts 20–30 minutes, after which sweating stops completely. However, this type of treatment often entails several undesirable phenomena and complications (including the formation of compensatory hyperhidrosis zones of other localizations), the incidence of which varies from 30 to 50%.

Intradermal botulinum toxin injections compare favorably with surgical treatment due to their high safety and good clinical efficacy. However, their effect is limited to about a year, after which the procedure must be repeated. Despite this limitation, in recent years, intradermal BoNT injection has become the most popular way to treat localized hyperhidrosis worldwide.

5.1. Mechanism of action

Unlike sebaceous glands (see Part III, chapter 4), sweat glands are controlled by the autonomic nervous system and respond to ACh released from the endings of autonomic neurons by increasing sweat production.

The structure of the cholinergic synapse between the nerve terminal and the sweat cell and the mechanism of signal transduction (ACh) are similar to those observed at the neuromuscular synapse (see Part I, chapter 1). It is therefore not surprising that botulinum toxin, having the capacity to block the release of the signaling mediator, is used to treat autonomic disorders associated with local cholinergic hyperactivity, such as:

- Hyperhidrosis (excessive sweating)
- Hypersalivation (increased salivation)
- Hyperlacrimation (excessive tear production)
- Erythrophobia (excessive and uncontrollable facial blushing in social or performance situations)

Although inconvenient to the individual, the latter three conditions are not aesthetic problems. On the other hand, hyperhidrosis significantly impacts a person's appearance and self-perception, which is why dermatologists may hear their patients complain of excessive sweating. With botulinum therapy, modern dermatologists can provide expert help to these individuals.

5.2. Clinical aspects

BoNT/A can treat all types of localized hyperhidrosis — both primary and secondary, including rare conditions such as hyperhidrosis of the face, head, and groin area. Compensatory hyperhidrosis never occurs after the procedure.

The skin in the treatment area should be prepared: in the axillary regions, it is recommended to shave all body hair, and in the foot area, a pedicure should be performed to eliminate hyperkeratosis (Vlahovic T.C., 2016).

Before BoNT/A injection, a Minor test is performed to clarify the size of the area affected by increased sweating.

Intradermal BoNT injection is quite painful, so anesthesia is mandatory. Topical anesthetic is applied one hour before the procedure. If additional anesthesia is required during the procedure, lidocaine spray can be used. When treating hyperhidrosis in the palms and feet, particularly in pain-sensitive patients or children, conduction anesthesia of the median, ulnar, and tibial nerves may be used. However, this is rarely done in practice.

The BoNT/A dose depends on the severity of hyperhidrosis and the size of the treated area; in men, the dose is usually higher — sometimes 1.5–2 times — compared to women. The drug is injected intradermally with an insulin syringe, spacing the injection points 1.5–2 cm apart. The number of injection points for one typical area (palm, foot, armpit, forehead) varies from 10 to 30. Injections are repeated as needed, with at least three-month intervals between applications.

The effect of "drying" the treated areas typically manifests after 2–3 days. It peaks in a week and is retained longer than when acting on neuromuscular connections — from 4–8 months to a year.

Small hematomas and soreness at the injection points may be observed in the treatment area for two days after the procedure. Still, they quickly disappear and do not require additional treatment. No adverse reactions occur if the injection technique and the recommended dosages are followed.

Hyperhidrosis in menopausal women is one of the most common reasons for seeking medical help. In this case, it is secondary or symptomatic and manifests in attacks of diffuse sweating, whereby the head, face, neck, back, and other body parts become wet. These events are usually accompanied by other autonomic symptoms such as heart palpitations, shortness of breath and rapid breathing, restlessness and anxiety, shivering and chills that progress to hot flashes, etc. In treating this form of hyperhidrosis, priority is given to the therapy aimed at the underlying condition (which should be prescribed by a gynecologist–endocrinologist or neurologist). Injectable botulinum therapy is not a generally accepted indication for this problem since there is widespread excessive sweating of almost the entire body surface. However, intradermal BoNT/A injections in excessive sweating on the face are possible. This practice can be compared to the intradermal injection of BoNT/A for treating facial erythrophobia (Park J.K. et al., 2022).

Limitations of this treatment are possible adverse events associated with the relaxing effect of the drug on mimic muscles, which may manifest as disorders of facial expression and articulation, especially when BoNT/A is administered in the middle and lower thirds of the face. Still, once the patient is informed about possible side effects and agrees to the procedure, it is possible to use this method as a part of complex therapy of the underlying disease. Another argument in support of botulinum therapy is the expected smoothing of expression lines in the injection areas, especially if indicated (e.g., in patients with pronounced marionette wrinkles). The peculiarities of administration are small doses of BoNT, strictly intradermal injections, and bilateral and symmetrical administration (to avoid facial asymmetry).

In contrast to menopausal hyperhidrosis, where botulinum therapy is considered an adjunctive treatment, for individuals affected by gustatory sweating, it is the method of choice (O'Neill J.P. et al., 2008; Fiedler L.S., Burk F., 2024). Intradermal BoNT injections result in a significant and persistent reduction of the sweating area without substantial adverse events. In some cases, remission can last for several years.

Résumé

Intradermal BoNT injection significantly improves the quality of life of patients suffering from autonomic nervous system disorders of various etiologies and severity, including localized forms of hyperhidrosis, which are included in the registered indications for injectable botulinum therapy.

The advantages of botulinum therapy are simplicity of administration, the ability to inject the drug into any body area, the rapid onset and duration of the clinical effect, and safety, proven by many years of international experience in BoNT use. The treatment has a persistent, pronounced clinical effect and allows patients to discontinue other drug and non-drug treatment methods and, in some cases, avoid surgery (Karamfilov T. et al., 2000; Nawrocki S., Cha J., 2020).

Chapter 6
Hair loss

Skincare specialists sometimes hear their patients complain about hair loss (alopecia), although this is not the main reason for their visit. Instead, it is information that patients share in confidence, expecting advice rather than a specific treatment. They turn to a dermatologist for that purpose, but a dermatologist without specialized training in trichology cannot address this issue effectively. In modern times, although considered a section of dermatology, trichology has become a separate discipline. To become a certified trichologist, it is necessary to undergo training and receive appropriate credentials. Thus, dermatologists who have completed this qualification process can provide practical assistance to patients with hair problems.

Androgenetic alopecia (AGA) is not on the list of registered indications for botulinum therapy, but clinical observations are showing the therapeutic effect of BoNT (Singh S. et al., 2017; Zhou Y. et al., 2020).

6.1. Androgenetic alopecia

AGA is a disorder that affects both men and women and manifests as hair thinning (to the point of absence) due to the progressive shrinkage of hair follicles. It is a non-scarring hair loss disorder, i.e., there is no previous skin damage or scarring in the hair loss area.

The AGA pathogenesis is still not fully understood. However, a signaling pathway triggered in hair follicle cells by dihydrotestosterone (DHT) via androgen receptors that leads to follicle miniaturization and hair loss is thought to play a key role in its development. DHT is produced in the dermal papilla from testosterone by the action of the enzyme 5α-reductase and then enters the follicle. The competitor of 5α-reductase is aromatase, which converts testosterone to estradiol.

Increased testosterone levels, increased 5α-reductase activity, and decreased aromatase activity along with increased androgen receptor expression, either in isolation or in combination, may cause AGA. The situation can worsen after acute stress or against the background of prolonged depression, in the presence of somatic or infectious diseases, or due to an unbalanced diet. Such etiologic diversity complicates the selection of AGA therapy in each specific case. How can BoNT help? Several hypotheses have been proposed.

One of the leading hypotheses on the effectiveness of BoNT in hair loss treatment attributes it to the relaxation of muscles in the forehead, occiput, temples, and surrounding the scalp (Zhou Y. et al., 2020). If contracted for an extended period, these muscles can disrupt subcutaneous blood flow and cause local hypoxia in the follicles. Under hypoxic conditions, the DHT-mediated signaling pathway is activated, leading to hair loss. Partial relaxation of these muscles by intramuscular BoNT injections may restore the blood supply and oxygenation to the hair follicles and reduce hair loss. While there is no reliable evidence to support this perspective, because headaches are intense stressors that can provoke massive hair loss, hair growth will normalize once the pain is over, and thus, the stress lessens.

Another hypothesis links the BoNT action to its ability to inhibit the production of TGF-β1 in dermal papilla cells (Shon U. et al., 2020). TGF-β1 is considered one of the key players in the development of AGA because it suppresses the growth of hair follicle epithelial cells. DHT stimulates TGF-β1 production and thus triggers a signaling pathway leading to hair follicle miniaturization and hair loss. Accordingly, Shon U. et al. (2020) argue that the results of their own immunofluorescence studies confirm the inhibition of TGF-β1 expression in the presence of BoNT, indicating that BoNT should be injected intradermally into the area of hair thinning.

6.2. Trichotillomania

Trichotillomania is a psychiatric disorder characterized by frequent, repeated, and irresistible urges to pull out hair from one's scalp, eyebrows, or other areas of the body. Engel E.R. and Ham J.A. (2023) described the case of a 30-year-old woman with a long history of trichotillomania who was resistant to behavioral therapy and medications. The patient also suffered from chronic migraines and was prescribed botulinum therapy for headache relief. The botulinum therapy was successful, and the headaches decreased significantly. After completing botulinum therapy, the patient received 45 IU of onabotulinumtoxinA intradermally into the scalp, 5 IU per point. The patient reported marked improvement in her trichotillomania signs and symptoms, which resulted in hair regrowth as early as the first follow-up visit 12 weeks post-treatment initiation. Treatment effects were maintained, and additional hair regrowth was observed at the 1-year post-treatment visit, by which point four treatment cycles had been completed.

Résumé

The feasibility of botulinum therapy for hair loss treatment is being explored, but we will have to wait for some time before practical recommendations can be made. Nonetheless, published systematic reviews point to optimistic conclusions, even if they show positive trends rather than statistically significant results (English R.S. Jr, Ruiz S., 2022; Nassar A. et al., 2022).

Yes, it has been observed that botulinum therapy can reduce hair loss in cases of AGA, but this does not mean that such treatment would benefit all patients. To develop treatment regimens with predictable results or, conversely, to abandon this type of therapy (such proposals are also expressed), it is necessary to understand the molecular and cellular mechanisms of BoNT action (Carloni R. et al., 2020). Let us hope that the knowledge we need will be available soon.

For more detailed information on hair health, see the *Hair Care in Cosmetic Dermatology & Skincare Practice* book.

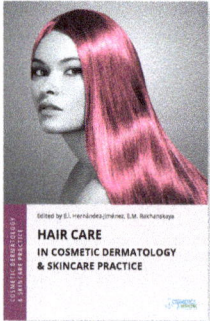

Edited by E.I. Hernández-Jiménez, S.M. Bachanskaya

HAIR CARE
IN COSMETIC DERMATOLOGY
& SKINCARE PRACTICE

Part IV

Combining botulinum therapy with aesthetic treatments

Modern aesthetic medicine offers patients a wide range of services provided in facilities with a medical license. Nonetheless, energy-based treatments (physiotherapy), minimally invasive injections, and chemical peeling remain the most popular, and these treatment modalities allow us to successfully, safely, and quickly correct age-related skin changes and maintain the achieved results. However, two questions must be addressed before combining treatments:

1. Is it safe?
2. Is it pathogenetically justified?

Only if both questions are answered in the affirmative can we develop optimal protocols for treatment regimens and establish appropriate intervals between treatments. Several important points should be considered in this context:

1. Mechanisms for developing certain effects when using specific device-based and injection techniques. This is necessary to identify common application points and to analyze the nature of the effects produced.
2. The level and nature of direct and indirect therapeutic effects and the potential for their positive or negative interaction when using a set of methods.

In this part, we will discuss the possibilities of combining injectable botulinum therapy with the most popular methods in solving aesthetic problems.

Chapter 1
Botulinum therapy and energy-based modalities

In complex programs, at the first stage, usually non-invasive low-energy physiotherapeutic treatments are performed, which prepare the skin for further manipulations. These procedures improve lymphatic drainage and microcirculation, intensify cellular and tissue metabolic processes, thicken the dermal matrix, and relieve inflammation. Prepared skin has a higher reparative potential and recovers faster and better after subsequent injections or high-energy device-based treatments.

Physiotherapy is often prescribed during rehabilitation. It prevents congestion and edema, reduces inflammation, and stimulates cell metabolism and healing processes.

1.1. Aims of physiotherapy in combination with botulinum therapy

The actual aim is to develop ways to enhance and prolong the clinical effect of botulinum therapy because frequently administered injections will significantly increase the cost while potentially provoking an immune response with the formation of antibodies, causing partial or complete insensitivity to treatment. This will not be critical for those receiving botulinum therapy for aesthetic indications. However, a decreased effectiveness can cause significant problems for a patient with a medical indication.

It has been established that a more pronounced and persistent myorelaxant effect develops at maximal muscle contraction during the procedure with a sufficient intracellular concentration of calcium ions (and possibly potassium) under the influence of low temperatures. Calcium deficiency in the body is detected with a simple neurological test of latent tetany (the test is based on the Chvostek sign* — tapping the cheek between the zygomatic arch and the corner of the mouth at the exit point of the facial nerve causes lightning-fast contractions of the muscles of the mouth, nose, and the outer eye corners). Some practitioners recommend that the patient take calcium preparations with vitamin D for prophylactic purposes two weeks before the BoNT injection. Immediately before and after the injection, the injection area is cooled, and the patient is instructed to actively tense the muscles where BoNT was injected for 15–30 minutes after the procedure and further during the day. Similar effects can be achieved using some device-based methods.

At the other end of the scale is a diametrically opposite problem — finding ways to neutralize the myorelaxant effect in case of excessive relaxation of the target muscle or diffusion of the toxin and relaxation of non-target muscles. This is a rather tricky task since the cleavage of SNARE clasp complex proteins is irreversible. Synaptic transmission restoration occurs due to the axon's collateral branches (sprouting phenomenon, see Part I, chapter 1), and physiotherapeutic procedures can play a role in this process.

Thus, combining physiotherapy and botulinum therapy in integrated treatment programs does not aim to sum up the effects of individual influences but considers their synergism or antagonism.

1.2. Energy-based treatments affect the intensity and duration of BoNT-assisted myorelaxant effect

Based on the understanding of the process of chemical muscle denervation, it is possible to distinguish several mechanisms of physiotherapeutic action, which make it possible to accelerate sprouting and

---

*The Chvostek sign is a clinical sign that someone may have a low blood calcium level (a decreased serum calcium, called hypocalcemia). It manifests as abnormal twitching of muscles that are activated (innervated) by the facial nerve (also known as Cranial Nerve Seven or CNVII).

restore innervation or, conversely, to enhance the myorelaxant effect of BoNT/A. The manifestation of these diametrically opposite effects will depend on the sequence of procedures during treatment and is realized due to three main mechanisms:

1. Facilitation of synaptic impulse transmission (neuromyostimulation)
2. Accelerating neuron regeneration and the sprouting process
3. Stimulation of metabolic processes against the background of microcirculation improvement (regenerating, tropho-stimulating, vasoactive action)

Energy-based methods can also be divided into three groups depending on the predominant mechanism of action:

1. **Neuromyostimulation methods:** low-frequency magnetic therapy, microcurrent therapy, electromyostimulation
2. **Reparative and regenerative methods:** ultrasound therapy, low-intensity infrared/red laser (light) therapy (LLLT)
3. **Vasodilating, tropho-stimulating methods:** mechanical stimulation of tissues in combination with cyclic vacuum action, microcurrent therapy, galvanization, and drug electrophoresis with vasodilating drugs, low-frequency pulsed magnetic therapy

Let us elaborate on some of these treatment modes.

1.2.1. Electromyostimulation

Electromyostimulation (EMS) is based on applying electric current to excite or enhance the activity of motor nerves and the contraction of skeletal and smooth muscles. This effect can be achieved by pulsed low-frequency modulated current, the strength of which, as a rule, does not exceed 100 mA (for facial muscles —no more than 50 mA).

The use of pulsed currents is necessary because the sensitivity of the skin and skeletal muscles' nerve fibers, estimated by the excitation current's threshold strength, is about three times higher for pulsed than direct currents. When a pulsed current passes through tissues (at the moments of its rapid activation and interruption), the local concentration of ions near cell membranes changes, which triggers appropriate physiological reactions in the cells of excitable tissues (nervous and muscular). By causing motor excitation and muscle contraction, pulsed electric currents simultaneously reflexively increase blood and lymph circulation and affect the entire complex of metabolic processes in muscles and nerves.

Periodic exposure to electric current in a specific mode affects axon growth and sprouting. It is possible that artificial depolarization causes changes of adaptogenic character in myelinated nerve fibers and motor nerve endings and promotes the development of collaterals and the formation of new synapses. The effect of muscle contraction may be caused by the stimulation of ACh release from functioning synapses during rhythmic depolarization of the axon membrane, with some amount of mediator appearing on the denervated areas and binding to receptors on the postsynaptic membrane, triggering muscle fiber contraction. Trophic effects of EMS can be associated with the expansion of peripheral vessels and blood flow. Thus, after botulinum therapy (at least two weeks later), EMS administration will restore the neuromuscular transmission and muscle contractility.

However, there is another aspect: stimulation of nerves and muscle contractile activity enhances the internalization of BoNT into the neuron. This is why patients are asked to tense their muscles before injection. By administering EMS immediately **before** the botulinum procedure and/or in the first 20–30 min after the injection, it is possible to aggravate the blocking effect of the toxin in relation to neuromuscular conduction and enhancement of myorelaxation.

Due to the peculiarities of muscle structure and physiology, the EMS modes for facial and neck muscles differ from those used for skeletal muscles. EMS of facial musculature requires increased caution due to the high dynamism of mimic muscles. In case of incorrect exposure mode, excessive and prolonged excitatory stimulation of thin muscle fibers can cause functional neurons to overstress: muscle "fatigue" is clinically manifested by increased hypo- or hypertonus.

The modes of EMS also differ significantly depending on the state of the neuromuscular apparatus. Thus, chemical denervation of a muscle is accompanied by excitability disturbance. Electrodiagnostics (assessment of the functional state of nerves and muscles based on the determination of their response to electrical stimulation) is thus recommended for the objective evaluation of the neuromuscular apparatus excitability to select EMS parameters commensurate with the actual changes (Yutskovskaya Y.A. et al., 2011).

EMS performed before the botulinum therapy procedure or within 20–30 minutes after injections will enhance the toxin's myorelaxant action.

Administration of EMS two weeks after botulinum therapy will result in accelerated recovery of neuromuscular conduction. This effect can be considered therapeutic in case of adverse events associated with spreading the toxin's myorelaxant action to non-target muscles or excessive relaxation of target muscles. On the other hand, it would be undesirable if adequate BoNT-assisted results were attained.

1.2.2. Microcurrent therapy

Microcurrent therapy is based on modulated pulsed currents of low strength (10–800 μA) and low intensity with different frequency characteristics. Unlike EMS, microcurrent therapy does not cause visible muscle contraction. It restores atrophied muscle fibers by normalizing intracellular processes and relieving muscle spasms. Fibrillation (i.e., rapid random contractions, "twitching") of smooth muscles of arterioles and superficial muscles of the skin caused by short electrical impulses activates metabolic processes and improves tissue tropism. Due to the resorption of edema, blood flow to ischemic tissue areas improves, and tactile sensitivity increases.

It is assumed that microcurrent therapy stimulates potential-dependent ion channels in the cell, causing therapeutic effects. Under the action of microcurrents, sodium and potassium ions are redistributed, leading to a change in membrane potential. Such "reverse" polarity lasts approximately 1–2 ms for epithelial cells and 3–5 ms for skeletal muscle cells. During this time, divalent cations, particularly calcium, enter the cell, generating a powerful physiological signal that triggers a cascade of intracellular reactions.

Microcurrent therapy performed **before** BoNT/A injections will not enhance the toxin's myorelaxant effect. However, if performed **after** botulinum therapy, it will promote sprouting and restore neuromuscular transmission.

> Microcurrent therapy performed before BoNT/A injections helps normalize muscle tone and does not affect the effectiveness of botulinum therapy.
>
> If microcurrent therapy is performed after botulinum treatment, it helps to level the BoNT effect by accelerating the restoration of neuromuscular transmission. This outcome can be considered favorable when the BoNT/A impact has spread to non-target muscles or in cases of excessive target muscle relaxation. In all other cases, microcurrent therapy in the areas of muscle chemodenervation should be avoided.

1.2.3. Galvanization and iontophoresis

Galvanization refers to applying a direct electric current of low strength (up to 50 mA) and low voltage (30–80 V). Depending on the state of the organism, the location of electrodes, and the current intensity, it can induce various physiological reactions of both local and general character.

In the skin, mainly in the cathode area, there is a release of biologically active substances — ACh, histamine, heparin, prostaglandins, endorphins, and factors that cause dilation of the vascular lumen (NO and endothelin). Under the action of these substances, hyperemia develops, which contributes to improving metabolism and accelerating redox processes. This has a resorptive effect and serves as a source of reflex irritation and accelerated epithelization of wounds and trophic ulcers. The galvanic current stimulates metabolism and triggers the activity of sebaceous and sweat glands.

Using galvanic current for transdermal drug administration (iontophoresis, syn.: electrophoresis) results in a high concentration of biologically active substances involved in nerve fiber regeneration, such as vitamins and vasodilators.

Galvanization before BoNT/A administration will not significantly affect the clinical effect; when performed after BoNT/A, it may weaken it and reduce its duration.

Prior to BoNT/A injections, calcium iontophoresis in the intended intervention zone may increase the efficacy of botulinum therapy. Iontophoresis of neurotropic vitamins and vasodilators helps restore neuromuscular conduction and can thus be beneficial in lessening the adverse events after botulinum therapy.

1.2.4. Low-intensity pulsed magnetic therapy

Low-frequency pulsed magnetic field (PMF) has a rather effective and, at the same time, gentle neurostimulating effect. Unfortunately, procedures involving PMF are not widely used in cosmetic dermatology. Still, their application is widespread in recovery programs after plastic surgeries to accelerate the healing of chronic wounds, trophic ulcers, burns, and keloid scars. Clinical studies also confirm the effectiveness of magnetic therapy in treating slow fractures, as well as for healing tendons and skin.

Magnetic therapy can also be used for remote (contactless) muscle stimulation (magnetic myostimulation). Namely, with the help of powerful PMF, inducing eddy currents in tissues at a depth of 4–6 cm, it is possible to cause selective contraction of both skeletal muscles and smooth muscles of vessels and internal organs. The action of magnetic fields on the neuromuscular apparatus also manifests in increased muscular endurance, thereby mitigating local and general fatigue conditions.

PMF increases the speed of impulse conduction along intact nerve fibers, increases their excitability, and causes rhythmic contraction of skeletal muscle myofibrils (magnetic stimulation). Perineural edema is also reduced, local blood flow is activated, and metabolism and regeneration are stimulated. Myelination processes, increased nerve trunk conductivity, lymph and blood circulation normalization, as well as improved axonal transport and synaptic transmission, contribute to restoring the neuromuscular apparatus's function. PMF has a significant anti-edematous and trophic effect and a pronounced neurostimulation effect.

An essential advantage of the method is the unlimited propagation of the magnetic field in space. As the PMF generator gets farther away, its influence weakens considerably but has no final boundaries. For the clinician, this means that it is possible to affect deep muscles, such as those of the eye, which are involved in developing serious complications of botulinum therapy, such as diplopia, strabismus, and others.

Low-intensity magnetic therapy is recommended when it is necessary to attenuate the myorelaxant effect of BoNT and accelerate the recovery of neuromuscular transmission.

1.2.5. Ultrasound therapy

For therapeutic proposes, special devices that generate ultrasound waves in a conical beam are used. Like any biological tissue, skin is a heterogeneous system comprising different structures (media) with different acoustic conductivity characteristics. In the transition of ultrasound from one medium to another, waves refract and/or reflect. Specifically, the refraction of ultrasound waves occurs at the boundary of epidermis/dermis and subcutaneous fat/muscle. Subcutaneous fat has the lowest absorption capacity, while it is the highest in muscles, nerves, and bone tissue. Energy absorption increases at the boundary of different tissues.

Therapeutic ultrasound vibrations regulate muscle tone, cause reflex vascular dilation, enhance capillary blood supply, and improve venous outflow. Owing to these effects, ultrasound is frequently used to accelerate wound healing. Although the subtle mechanisms of this effect remain unexplored, according to Maeshige N. et al. (2011), an increase in the expression of smooth muscle alpha-actin (α-SMA) and TGF-β is the basis for accelerating the healing of chronic wounds under the influence of ultrasound. Kruse D.E. et al. (2008) similarly noted an increase in the synthesis of one of the leading heat shock proteins* — Hsp70 — within the skin area treated with ultrasound, which persisted for four days.

As for the effect on nerve endings, it has been shown that ultrasound increases synaptic activity and activates neurovegetative processes (Ulashchik V.S., Timoshenko O.N., 2008).

> Ultrasound therapy contributes to the restoration of neuromuscular conduction. Thus, such procedures after botulinum therapy can theoretically reduce its effectiveness.

1.2.6. Low-level laser (light) therapy

Low-level laser (light) therapy (LLLT) with a wavelength in the 650–900 nm range (red and infrared [IR] regions of the spectrum) is actively used in the rehabilitation period after surgery, as well as in the treatment of subacute and chronic inflammatory diseases of the skin and subcutaneous tissue, large non-healing wounds and trophic ulcers, burns and frostbite, pruritic dermatoses, and furunculosis.

Several hypotheses have been proposed to explain the biophysical and physiological mechanisms underlying the impact of photobiomodulation on cells and tissues. While these hypotheses are based on a large body of experimental evidence (Hamblin M., 2006), the mitochondrial hypothesis remains the most popular. It posits that LLLT targets cytochrome c-oxidase, accelerating electron transport along the mitochondrial respiratory chain during oxidative phosphorylation (Karu T., 2010).

According to another hypothesis, low-level red and IR irradiation can provoke photochemical reactions such as lipid photooxidation in cell membranes, photoreactivation of superoxide dismutase (SOD), or photolysis of some substances with NO release. As a result, ROS is

---

*Heat shock proteins act as chaperones, i.e., they repair disorders in the stacking of other proteins. These "repairer" proteins are produced during cell damage caused by various stresses, and their synthesis allows the cell to tolerate stressors regardless of their nature. Production of these proteins is the basis for the increasing organism's resistance to unfavorable environmental factors.

released in a more significant amount, and oxidative stress occurs in the cell, forcing it to mobilize its defense and detoxification systems (Vladimirov Y.A. et al., 2004).

While these and other explanations for the LLLT photomodulatory effect remain scientifically unverified, the clinical impact of promoting tissue repair and increasing its resistance to stressors remains undeniable.

LLLT promotes nerve regeneration and restoration of conduction. LLLT in the area of muscle chemodenervation after botulinum therapy can weaken the effect of myorelaxation and is therefore inadvisable.

1.2.7. Mechanical stimulation

In demand in clinical practice, the mechanical method combines massaging skin tissues with rollers and pulsed vacuum. This activates blood flow and lymphatic drainage, improving trophic processes and reducing swelling.

Performing such procedures on the face can theoretically accelerate the recovery of contractility in muscles that were relaxed by botulinum therapy, but the effect will not be significant.

1.2.8. Thermal stimulation

Some practitioners believe that any effect associated with tissue heating — RF lifting, broadband pulsed light (IPL) therapy, and laser treatment, including fractional mode — will reduce the effectiveness of botulinum therapy. Indeed, BoNT is thermolabile, but it can be inactivated only by deep warming of skin tissues in the area of intradermal and subcutaneous injections in the first 30–60 min.

In practice, when performing the above procedures, we obtain controlled, limited-in-depth, short-term heating that does not extend to the level of muscle structures and has neither the neuromyostimulating nor sufficient thermal effect needed to inactivate BoNT.

Some increase in subcutaneous blood flow in the heating zone may have a tropho-stimulating effect not only at the level of dermis and hypodermis but also in nearby anatomical structures, indirectly accelerating the sprouting processes. However, considering the long interval between device-based procedures (1–3 weeks) and the short duration of hyperemia, it can be assumed that such an effect is minimal and clinically insignificant.

Considering heat-based procedures in general, we can say that their "influence" on the effects of BoNT is associated exclusively with the activation of the microcirculatory channel and trophic processes. These phenomena are most pronounced with deep heating of tissues during a visit to a sauna, including the IR modality. However, as such effects occur infrequently, a pronounced weakening of the impact of botulinum therapy should not be expected.

Procedures associated with local tissue heating (RF lifting, IPL, non-ablative laser treatment, including fractional mode) performed before or after BoNT injections do not significantly affect the efficacy of botulinum therapy.

1.2.9. Other physical modalities

Microdermabrasion, gas-liquid peeling, and non-invasive oxygen mesotherapy work mainly at the epidermis level and cause relatively weak indirect trophic effects in the superficial muscular aponeurotic system (SMAS). There is no antagonistic influence on the myorelaxant effect of botulinum therapy.

Microdermabrasion, gas-liquid peeling, and non-invasive oxygen mesotherapy are safe skincare treatments that don't interfere with muscle chemodenervation by BoNT.

Résumé

A rational combination of BoNT injections and physiotherapeutic techniques allows practitioners to perform several tasks:

- Potentiate the myorelaxant effect of BoNT/A without increasing the dose (calcium iontophoresis performed before the procedure, EMS performed immediately before and/or in the first 20–30 min after BoNT/A administration).
- Contribute to the early resolution of possible transient adverse effects of botulinum therapy without reducing its therapeutic effect (massage in the lymphatic drainage program for edema after BoNT/A injections in the periorbital area).
- Weaken the myorelaxant effect of BoNT/A by stimulation of sprouting in case of hypercorrection or BoNT diffusion into non-target muscles (EMS two weeks after injections, low-frequency electromagnetic field application, microcurrent therapy, iontophoresis of neurotropic drugs, LLLT).

Considering the mechanisms of neuromuscular transmission restoration and the nature of a physiotherapeutic impact (direct or indirect), the antagonistic effect is the greatest for neuromyostimulating modalities, intermediate for reparative-regenerative modalities, and minimal for tropho-stimulating modalities (**Table IV-1-1**).

Accordingly, when developing complex treatment regimens for involutional skin changes, botulinum therapy can be combined with skin tightening treatments (photorejuvenation, RF lifting), non-invasive oxygen mesotherapy, microdermabrasion, and gas-liquid peeling.

When prescribing techniques such as roller massage combined with vacuum and LLLT, the patient should be informed of the possible slight reduction in the BoNT/A effect.

Microcurrent therapy and ultrasound therapy should be administered only in neighboring anatomical areas. EMS, magnetic stimulation, and galvanization should be performed only in exceptional cases or in topographical areas sufficiently far from BoNT injection sites.

Understanding the mechanisms of action of the applied modalities, objective evaluation of the skin condition, its constitutional and age-related features, and reasonable combination of different impacts allow

Table IV-1-1. Compatibility of botulinum therapy with physiotherapy modalities in one anatomical zone

PHYSIOTHERAPY MODALITY	COMPATIBILITY WITH BONT	EXPLANATION
EMS	–	Neuromyostimulation
Microcurrent therapy	–	
Galvanization, iontophoresis	–	
Magnetic therapy	–	Clinically significant reparative and regenerative action against axon
LLLT	–	
Ultrasound therapy	–	
Roller massage with intermittent vacuum action	+/–	Prominent tropho-stimulantion
RF lifting	+	Clinically insignificant tropho-stimulatory mediated effect
Photorejuvenation (IPL)	+	
Oxygen mesotherapy (non-invasive)	++	Different depth of impact + no impact on axon regeneration
Microdermabrasion, gas-liquid peeling	++	

"–": do not combine; "+/–": the benefit of combination is not obvious; "+": can be combined; "++": combination is recommended

practitioners to obtain excellent clinical results and meet the patient's expectations (Karpova E.L., 2018).

For more detailed information on low-level energy-based methods, consult our *Microcurrent, Ultrasound, and LED Therapy in Cosmetic Dermatology & Skincare Practice* book.

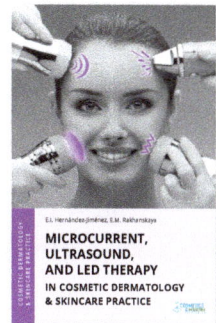

Chapter 2
Botulinum therapy and aesthetic injections

Combining botulinum therapy with aesthetic injections significantly expands its capabilities in dealing with age-related facial changes associated with increasing volume deficit and decreasing skin elasticity. Although such metamorphoses occur across the face and body, in some areas, they lead to the most pronounced aesthetic problems — deep wrinkles and folds, hollows under the eyes and in the temporal zone, flabby skin, ptosis, and lip flattening.

All these signs of aging are based on atrophy in the subcutaneous fat (decrease in the fat "cushion" volume) and dermis (decrease in hyaluronic acid and accumulation of damaged structural proteins). Active facial expressions and muscle hypertonus aggravate these processes. If their activity is reduced with BoNT, it is possible to minimize their contribution to age-related structural changes in the skin. However, this will not compensate for the volume deficit, will not restore the hyaluronic acid content, and will not replace worn collagen-elastin fibers with new ones.

What can be done to attain these effects? Obviously, botulinum therapy should be combined with other cosmetic injections (Landau M., 2006; Klein A.W., Fagien S., 2007; Goldman A., Wollina U., 2010; Wollina U., Payne C.R., 2010; Nanda S., Bansal S., 2013; Moon H. et al., 2021; Li K. et al., 2022).

2.1. BoNT and hyaluronic fillers

By implanting hyaluronic fillers into soft tissues, their internal volume is increased. This equalizes skin relief in wrinkles/folds and facilitates volumetric reshaping of the full face or its separate segments (eyebrows, nose, lips, chin). When hyaluronic fillers are combined with

BoNT, we can harmonize the face and emphasize its gender-specific features (Sundaram H. et al., 2016b).

This strategy is widely used in aesthetic medicine, as evident from many articles describing studies, clinical cases, and treatment protocols. For example, according to Beer K.R. et al. (2014), after the combined correction of periorbital and interbrow areas, 65% of patients speak about "excellent results" which cannot be attained with monotherapy. This is not surprising, given that when BoNT/A and hyaluronic filler are injected into one area, the effect of the filler is prolonged by limiting the pressure on the tissues (de Maio M., 2004) by almost 200% according to the observations of some specialists (Carruthers J., Carruthers A., 2001). Complex therapy is particularly effective in areas with high mimic activity: frontal, interbrow, and perioral. In some patients, regular BoNT/A injections reduce the extent of dynamic and static wrinkles (de Maio M., 2004; Nanda S., Bansal S., 2013). There is also the possibility of a positive impact of BoNT on dermal fibroblasts.

The preventive role of such a combination is also discussed in scientific literature. In areas with active facial expressions, fibrous strands are formed over time, connecting the dermis with SMAS and serving as the morphological basis for forming static wrinkles (Coleman K.R., Carruthers J., 2006). The ability of hyaluronic fillers to stimulate collagen production by fibroblasts has also been demonstrated (Wang F. et al., 2007).

Repeated BoNT/A and filler injections slow down facial involution. Moreover, with each subsequent injection, the required BoNT/A dose and filler volume can be reduced without losing efficacy. This is advantageous not only for safety reasons but also for attaining a more natural facial appearance (Coleman K.R., Carruthers J., 2006; Carruthers J. et al., 2008; Carruthers A. et al., 2010).

What should be considered when working in different areas of the face? What are their characteristic aesthetic problems? What are the main risks? We will dwell on these issues separately.

2.1.1. Upper third of the face

Botulinum therapy is the leading (and sometimes the only) treatment in this area, and filler injections can be an adjunct (de Maio M. et al., 2017a).

Horizontal wrinkles on the forehead

These wrinkles primarily bother women, but men seek correction at the stage when dynamic wrinkles turn into deep static furrows.

In most cases, BoNT/A injections can effectively smooth horizontal wrinkles without any undesirable consequences. In rare cases, after the procedure, eyebrow lowering or changes in their shape occur due to the redistribution of the activity of the levator (frontal) muscle and the depressors. Typically, this happens in aged patients who arbitrarily raise their eyebrows, trying to compensate for the overhanging of the upper eyelid. In young patients, however, timely and successfully performed botulinum therapy overcomes the mimic habit and reduces the dynamic pressure on the skin in this area.

Fillers can also correct horizontal forehead wrinkles. To avoid contouring, the "lightest" and high-plasticity filler should be chosen (**Fig. IV-2-1**).

Deep folds require a combination of two techniques: first, botulinum therapy is performed to relax the upper frontalis muscle, after which a small volume of hyaluronic filler is injected to smooth the wrinkles.

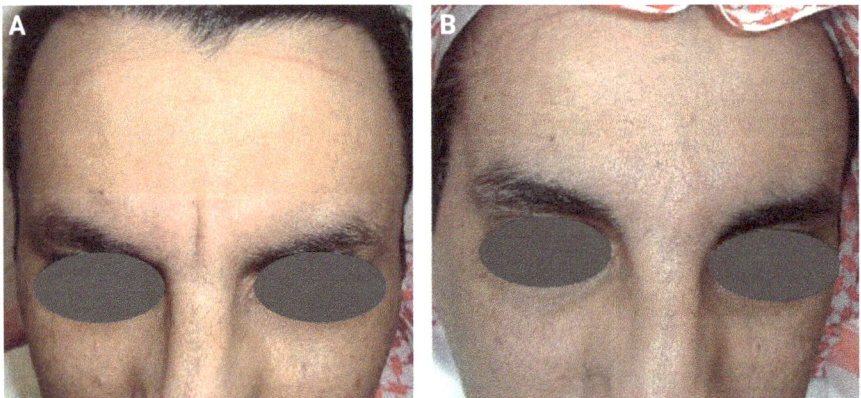

Figure IV-2-1. Excessive volume correction of the interbrow area due to difficulties in determining an adequate filler volume and botulinum therapy protocol: (A) before and (B) after combined treatment (adapted from Eleowa S.A., Zidan S.M., 2013)

Vertical creases in the interbrow area

In young patients, the vertical interbrow folds are dynamic, and BoNT/A monotherapy is performed to correct them and prevent the formation of static wrinkles in the future. An essential benefit of this strategy is that the patient's face no longer looks frowning and preoccupied, facilitating social communication.

In middle-aged patients, dynamic and static components can often be identified in the folds of the interbrow area. In this case, botulinum therapy will improve the appearance but will not fully equalize the skin topography (Nanda S., Bansal S., 2013). Combined therapy will give more prominent aesthetic results (**Fig. IV-2-2A,B**). It will also prolong

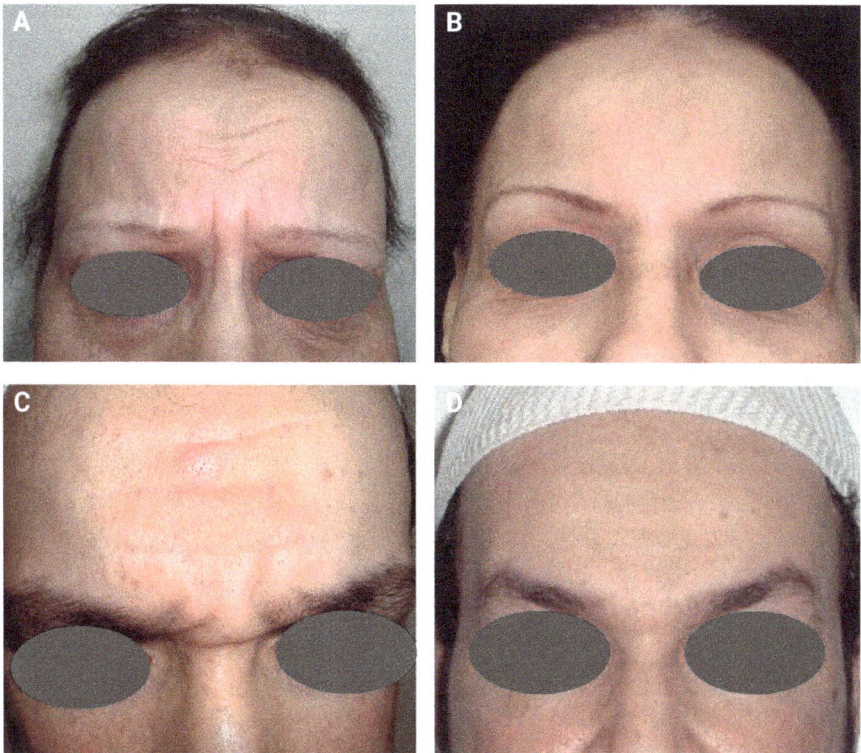

Figure IV-2-2. Interbrow fold correction with BoNT/A and filler injections (along with botulinum treatment in the forehead area): 50-year-old patient (A) before and (B) 180 days after the procedure; 42-year-old patient (C) before and (D) 360 days after the procedure (adapted from Eleowa S.A., Zidan S.M., 2013)

the filler's effect, which is administered minimally (Carruthers J., Carruthers A., 2001).

The last remark is fundamental, as it pertains to safety: the interbrow area belongs to the zones of increased risk of vascular complications, and the introduction of a minimal volume of filler prevents the emergence of compression-ischemic complications (Bosniak S. et al., 2006).

Initial planning of the two-stage combination therapy allows injections into the *corrugator supercilii* muscle* at medial points only, preventing significant divergence of the brow heads in patients who have previously experienced this undesirable phenomenon.

Horizontal line at the bridge of the nose

This line is caused by the increased tone of the *procerus* muscle, which lowers the nose's bridge. In most cases, BoNT/A injections solve this problem (**Fig. IV-2-2C,D**). Additional filler injection is allowed only if indicated.

Eyebrows

The eyebrows' position, shape, and mobility play a considerable role in the aesthetic perception of the face, including the ability of others to read one's emotions. There are precise gender specificities in the shape and position of the eyebrows. Age-related alterations often manifest in eyebrow lowering, which gives the female face a frowning, dissatisfied expression. On the other hand, this is beneficial for men because the low position of eyebrows emphasizes firmness and authority (Coleman K.R., Carruthers J., 2006).

BoNT/A injections raise the entire eyebrow (1–2 mm) or its lateral part (tail), thus modeling the shape. Filler injection in the eyebrow's tail allows the practitioner to create/emphasize the shape of the eyebrow in the form of a gull's wing. A convex area reflecting light under the eyebrow's tail also contributes to a younger appearance (Peskova I.V., 2014).

---

*The *corrugator supercilii* muscle is a small, narrow pyramidal facial muscle. It arises from the medial end of the superciliary arch and inserts into the deep surface of the eyebrow skin. It draws the eyebrow downward and medially, producing vertical "frowning" wrinkles in the forehead. It may be thought as the principal muscle in the facial expression of suffering. It also shields the eyes from strong sunlight.

2.1.2. Mid-face area

Contouring filler injections are often performed in this region (although there are exceptions). BoNT/A injections are an adjunctive treatment (de Maio M. et al., 2017b).

"Crow's feet"

The "crow's feet" in the outer eye corners are dynamic wrinkles, so botulinum therapy is a treatment of choice for correcting them. Extended wrinkles require an additional line of BoNT/A injections in the temporal region.

In wrinkles "descending" to the zygomatic region, there is a higher risk of neurotoxin diffusion into the zygomatic muscles with the subsequent development of functional disorders. In this case, either BoNT/A injections are performed superficially (intradermally), or downward wrinkles are corrected using hyaluronic fillers with high plasticity.

Fine lines on the cheeks

Botulinum therapy can be used to correct fine cheek wrinkles ("accordion wrinkles") (Mole B., 2012, 2014) (**Fig. IV-2-3**). However, the same wrinkles can be smoothed by mixed injections of native or stabilized hyaluronic acid; such treatment also increases the skin turgor.

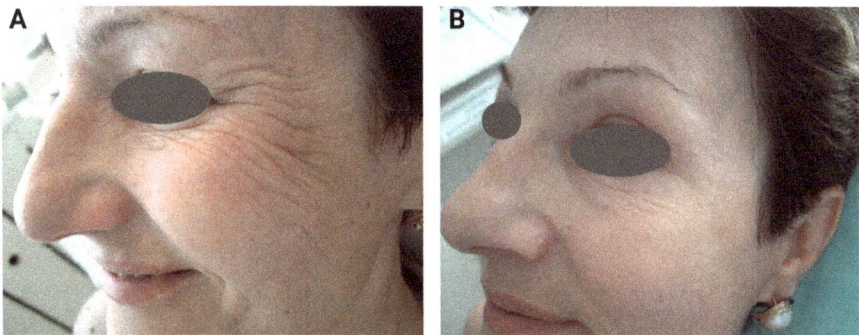

Figure IV-2-3. Correction of "accordion wrinkles" in the cheek area: (A) before and (B) two weeks after intradermal BoNT injection (adapted from Peskova I.V., 2014)

Furrows in the suborbital area

Deep furrows in the suborbital area can be a constitutional feature of skinny patients and/or be formed due to age-related fat atrophy and displacement and bone resorption in the eye socket area. The dark shadows make the furrows appear even more profound.

Subocular and nasolabial furrows are corrected by injecting filler into the deep layers of soft tissues (Karpova E.I., Gubanova E.I., 2010). Too convex lower eyelids (more typical for oriental faces) can be smoothed by a single BoNT/A injection along the mid-pupillary line 2–3 mm below the eyelash margin (Coleman K.R., Carruthers J., 2006). The correction of lower eyelid wrinkles is performed in the same way.

Perhaps, against the background of relaxation of the lower portion of the round eye muscle, it is possible to prevent the displacement of the filler under the muscle at its increased activity.

Volume loss in the cheek and cheekbone region

The cheek-maxillary region of a young face characteristically alternates between convex and depressed areas (smooth curves of the Oggi line). With age, due to the atrophy/redistribution of fat tissue and resorption of underlying bones, the face flattens, and so does the Oggi curve. Volumetric correction of the zygomatic and cheek areas allows the face to regain youthful relief. The procedure is successfully performed with relatively dense fillers, usually injected under the muscles.

Nose shape

The nasal tip can be raised by injecting BoNT/A into the depressor septum muscle (*m. depressor septi nasi*). Injections into the medial portion of the upper lip and wing muscle (*m. levator labii superioris alaequae nasi*) help reduce nose width and prevent the nostrils from flaring during facial expressions and articulation.

The filler injections correct the nose ridge (depressions, small humps) and, less often, the shape of the nose tip (this area is dangerous in terms of compression-ischemic complications).

Minimally invasive rhinoplasty is typically performed in several stages using both techniques.

2.1.3. Lower third of the face

The lower third of the face is a zone where combined therapy is predominantly used.

Lip shape

Lip contouring and volume correction are traditional indications for hyaluronic filler injections. However, if the upper lip needs to be increased in size without changing its volume, minimal doses of BoNT/A can be injected into points located along the red border (but away from the corners of the mouth).

Perioral wrinkles

The method for correcting perioral wrinkles is chosen after differential skin analysis. If "barcode" wrinkles are caused by solar elastosis or smoking, it is advisable to use hyaluronic fillers with high plasticity.

When wrinkles form against the background of increased tone of the circular muscles surrounding the mouth (*m. orbicularis oris*) and significantly worsen once the lips are pulled forward, correction is carried out with BoNT/A microdose injections in points several mm from the red border.

In patients whose profession necessitates prolonged and repetitive use of *orbicularis oris* muscles (singers, wind instrument players, teachers, interpreters, TV and radio commentators, etc.), botulinum therapy in this area is not recommended, and dermal fillers come to the forefront. Still, some patients may benefit from combined therapy.

"Marionette" wrinkles

Correcting "marionette" wrinkles can be challenging, as their emergence can be associated with different issues. If they result from the increased tone of muscles that lower the mouth corners, they are usually accompanied by the mouth corner lowering, and a deformation of the facial oval line by sagging checks. If so, the optimal correction technique is botulinum therapy (BoNT/A is injected into the muscles that lower the mouth corners and into the upper portion of the platysma). As an additional option, the fold can be reinforced with filler.

On the other hand, when the facial oval is sufficiently preserved and the mouth corners are in normal position, "marionette" wrinkles most likely arise due to the displacement of the soft tissue of the cheek, held by the mandibular ligament, medially downward. In this case, the method of choice is volumetric correction of the cheek-mandibular region, which will elevate the soft tissue mass and smooth the cheek–chin boundary. Botulinum therapy is performed more for preventive purposes: according to Le Louarn C. et al. (2007b), protrusion of fat tissue in the lower jaw area and the formation of "marionette" wrinkles are associated with hypertonus of some portions of the muscle lowering the corner of the mouth.

Lowered corners of the mouth

Combination therapy is preferable for correcting drooping mouth corners: along with BoNT/A injections, a filler is injected in the area under the lip commissures using a reinforcing or micro-bolus technique.

Face contour

Smoothing of the facial oval shape usually requires a combination of injections: BoNT/A to relax the mouth corners and platysma muscle, along with filler in the area of pronounced depressions along the mandibular margin (bolus injection or "fanning" reinforcement) (**Fig. IV-2-4**).

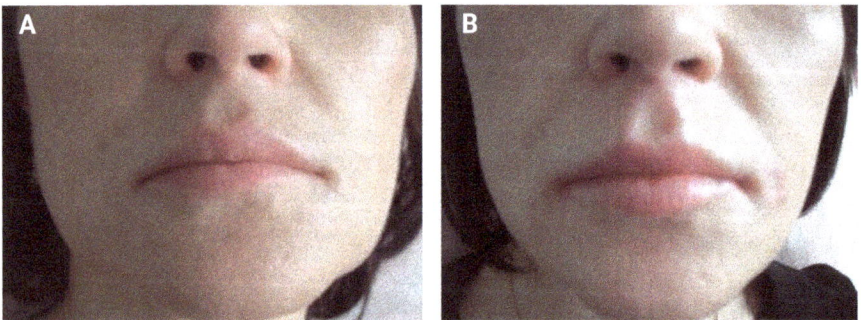

Figure IV-2-4. Patient, 50 years old. Combined correction of the facial oval line with BoNT/A and hyaluronic filler: (A) before and (B) after complex therapy (adapted from Peskova I.V., 2014)

2.1.4. Neck

In this zone, the choice of method is based on the identification of the leading problem:

- Tense platysma masses are corrected with BoNT/A injections
- Horizontal neck wrinkles are smoothed with BoNT/A and hyaluronic filler injections (Li Y. et al., 2022).

2.2. Can botulinum therapy and filler contouring be performed in one session?

Introducing BoNT and fillers in one session is possible when treating different anatomical zones.

However, when working in one anatomical zone, the procedures should be separated in time and performed in the following sequence:

1. Botulinum therapy is performed first. Hyaluronic filler, a highly hydrophilic material, changes tissue properties, possibly affecting BoNT/A diffusion. As previously noted, the predictability of the area of drug administration is the key to botulinum therapy's success.

2. It is recommended that the filler be injected two weeks after BoNT/A injections, which coincides with the peak of toxin action in most patients. In this case, the clinical picture can be evaluated, and the lowest necessary filler volume should be used for additional correction.

When performing combined treatment in the periorbital area, the interval between treatments may need to be increased even further. The relaxation of the circular muscle of the eye makes lymphatic drainage in this area more complex, and edema may occur after hydrophilic filler injection. After a few weeks, adequate drainage is restored, and the filler can be injected.

Why do many experts advise against performing a one-zone correction with BoNT/A and fillers on the same day? There are several reasons:

- The naked eye will determine the required filler volume without considering the leveling of skin relief due to myorelaxation.
- After filler injection, tissue properties change, and hemorrhages may form, possibly affecting the diffusion of the toxin.
- Skin cooling is used before and after the filler injection to increase the procedure's comfort and prevent hemorrhage; however, this technique can decrease the effectiveness of botulinum therapy.
- Before and after botulinum therapy, active facial expression is recommended for several hours, whereas mimic rest is required after the filler injection to prevent displacement of the injected material.

2.3. BoNT and other injectable preparations

In addition to hyaluronic fillers used for volumetric contouring, injectable cosmetic dermatology products include preparations for intradermal injection designed to improve skin quality — **mesococktails, biorevitalizants, platelet-rich plasma (PRP)** preparations. These aqueous solutions contain water-soluble biologically active substances in various amounts and combinations. The solutions are injected intradermally using the nappage technique through multiple punctures, treating large areas simultaneously. The skin reacts to extensive trauma with erythema and edema and may remain in this state for several days. Botulinum therapy is performed in advance (at least two weeks before the procedure) or postponed until after the swelling has completely subsided.

Post-treatment swelling is especially pronounced in biorevitalization — this method is based on the multiple intradermal introductions of high-molecular-weight native hyaluronic acid, which attracts water and creates a kind of hydro-reserve in the skin. Therefore, when combining botulinum therapy and biorevitalization, it is essential to allow for adequate intervals between procedures. An algorithm of combined treatment with BoNT and biorevitalizants proposed by Parsagashvili E.Z. (2010) can be consulted for this purpose. Against the background of facial muscle relaxation, especially in the periorbital area, fluid drainage worsens, and edema may occur. Introducing a hydrophilic substance — high-molecular-weight native hyaluronic acid — can aggravate the situation. Therefore, it is better to conduct botulinum therapy at the end of the biorevitalization course. By waiting 2–3 weeks after the last session, we can ensure that exogenous hyaluronic acid will no longer be present in the skin, while the effect of its action will remain. If additional biorevitalization procedures are required, they should be performed 3–4 months after BoNT introduction.

Biodegradable threads are implanted in the skin for lifting purposes. They create a framework that provides rapid skin tensioning and smoothing. As the material biodegrades over time, bands of fibrosis are formed in the skin in place of the thread, which causes the lifting effect to persist for some time. Botulinum therapy is often preceded by thread lifting, which is performed after the maximal impact of relaxation of target muscles has been noted (Surovykh S.V. et al., 2012).

If long "ribs of rigidity" are created with the help of threads and lifting occurs mainly due to frame tension, by introducing a gel preparation with **calcium hydroxyapatite** microparticles, the skin is compacted over a large area. Calcium hydroxyapatite stimulates collagen production by fibroblasts, so after its complete resorption, the skin is tighter (Eviatar J. et al., 2015). Botulinum therapy is performed before calcium hydroxyapatite injection (Almeida de A.T. et al., 2019).

Mesotherapy, biorevitalization, and PRP therapy often become the third component in a complex anti-aging program, complementing the "BoNT + fillers" and "BoNT + threads" combinations (Braccini F. et al., 2010). They help ameliorate the epidermal signs of aging associated with pigmentation disorders (age spots, uneven tone) and keratinization alterations (keratosis, roughness, superficial fine lines, dullness) while also normalizing the skin water balance by stimulating hyaluronic acid production and increasing the regenerative potential. As a result, the skin tone becomes lighter and more even, fine lines become less noticeable, and the skin looks fresher and more youthful (**Fig. IV-2-5**).

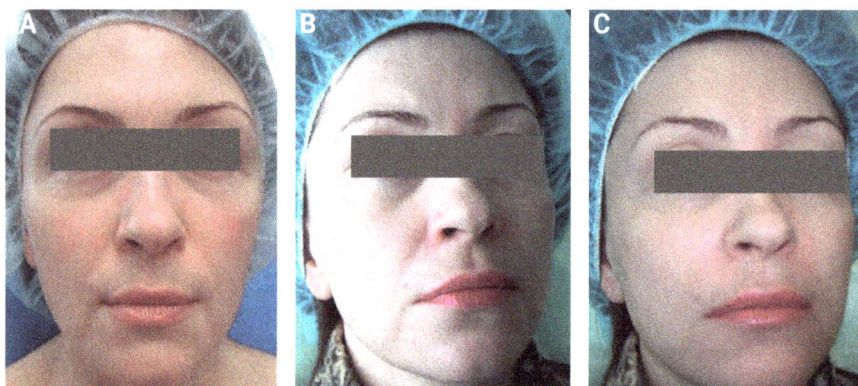

Figure IV-2-5. Patient, 45 years old: (A) before and (B) after botulinum therapy of the upper third of the face, (C) after hyaluronic filler injection in nasolabial folds and "marionette" wrinkles and biorevitalization (adapted from Peskova I.V., 2014)

Résumé

Long-term clinical practice confirms the necessity and possibility of including botulinum therapy in complex programs to prevent and correct age-related changes. Each method has its own advantages and limitations, indications and contraindications, and botulinum therapy is not an exception (Carruthers J. et al., 2008; Anand C., 2016; Carruthers J. et al., 2016; Fabi S.G. et al., 2016).

The choice and sequence of procedures should be pathogenetically justified and based on an understanding of the mechanisms of action of each method used, as well as their potential interactions. It should consider the patient's needs, gender, age, health status, and aging morphotype. In addition, the physician must have in-depth knowledge of the methods that will be applied and the capacity to assess their suitability for a particular patient. After all, the main goal is to emphasize the best aspects of the patient's face, ensuring that both the physician and the patient will get satisfaction from a job well done.

Botulinum toxin — there is only one! This is not simply a well-sounding phrase, but a balanced conclusion based on the uniqueness and selectivity of the action of this substance, predictability of its effects, high safety, and a wide range of clinical applications.

Part V

"Botox-like" skincare products

Injection is the most effective way to deliver BoNT to the target. Nevertheless, several aspects (in addition to contraindications and potential adverse events) should be considered before offering it to patients.

An important psychological aspect is related to the patient's attitude towards injections. There are people for whom the upcoming injection is a cause of great stress and who may refuse the procedure just because it requires an injection, while for others, the fact that "toxin is poison" also plays a role.

Needle pricks can cause adverse reactions, such as flu-like symptoms, muscle weakness, headache, facial pain, and redness. These reactions can partly be explained as a response to psychological stress, but it is possible to have hypersensitivity to point pain (individual characteristics of the sensory apparatus).

Topical BoNT may be the solution. It could cause less pronounced muscle relaxation, rendering it potentially safer in areas where muscles are susceptible to even small doses of toxin. A strong argument in favor of topical BoNT is avoiding complications associated with drug overdose and/or incorrect identification of injection points, which can lead to paralysis of the treated area lasting several months.

Topical application is comfortable and can be performed at home. However, the medical community dealing with botulinum therapy is against the free sale of external medicines containing BoNT. This caution is due to the risk of uncontrolled and inappropriate use, which could harm patient's health and undermine general confidence in the method.

Since BoNT is a rather large protein molecule, it cannot be expected to overcome the barrier structures of the *stratum corneum* on its own. However, in addition to targeted transdermal transfer, the developers of topical preparations face another task — stabilizing unstable BoNT, which is very sensitive to external conditions and is quickly inactivated in a medium other than the physiological solution.

In addition, as BoNT is a poison, its use in cosmetics is prohibited. Thus, natural BoNT is unsuitable for cosmetic formulations and must be replaced by a non-drug substance with a different chemical nature but similar clinical effects (e.g., "Botox-like" synthetic peptides) or a modification of natural BoNT approved for cosmetic use. These are the two ways the development of cosmetics "with botulinum toxin effect" was approached, which eventually culminated in the appearance of cosmetic products with unique properties on the market.

1.1. Mimicking the action of botulinum toxin

"Botox-like" peptides were the first to enter the market. Synthetic peptides act as the active ingredient in these products, as they can block the signal transmission from nerve endings to muscle fibers (**Fig. V-1**).

First on the list of "Botox-like" peptides is Argireline® peptide (INCI: Acetyl Hexapeptide-8). Having appeared in the early 2000s, it quickly gained popularity — today it can be found in many cosmetic products aimed at combating expression lines. The six amino acids of Argireline® replicate a fragment of the SNAP-25, which is necessary for binding the synaptic vesicle of the axon to the presynaptic membrane. In the axon, Argireline® competes with the SNAP-25 protein and is incorporated instead into the temporary SNARE protein complex — this complex is formed from several membrane proteins just before the vesicle binds to the membrane and is required for successful exocytosis. A defective complex cannot provide the necessary contact between the vesicle and the membrane, thus precluding the release of mediator into the synaptic cleft. This means the muscle does not receive a signal to contract and remains relaxed. Another synthetic peptide called SNAP-8™ (INCI: Acetyl Glutamyl Heptapeptide-1) acts

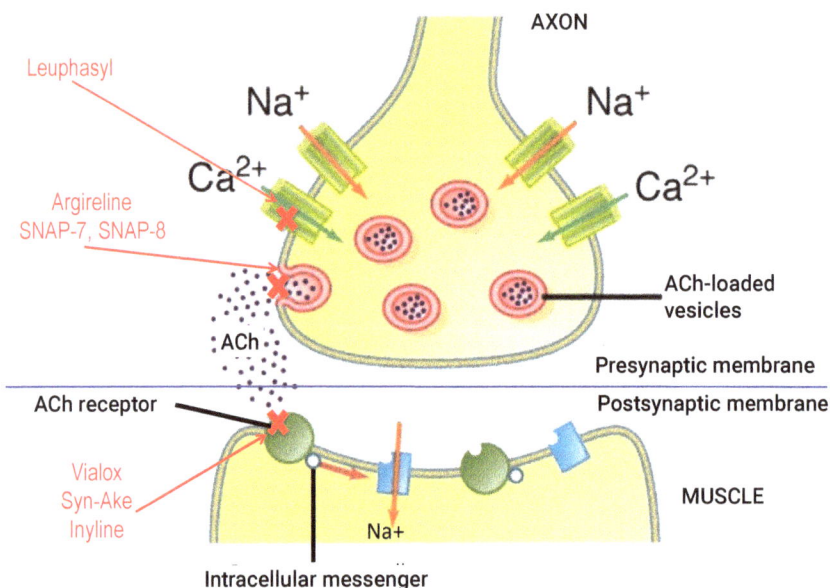

Figure V-1. Intracellular targets of "Botox-like" peptides

Cosmetic "Botox-like" peptides inhibit but do not destroy:

- **Argireline** (INCI: Acetyl Hexapeptide-8), **SNAP-7, SNAP-8** – sequences of 6–8 amino acids representing a fragment of SNAP-25 protein. Competes with it for a place in the SNARE complex.

- **Leuphasyl** (INCI: Pentapeptide-18) mimics the action of enkephalin. It reduces neuronal excitation by inhibiting the flow of calcium ions across the membrane and reduces Ca^{2+}-dependent mediator release.

- **Vialox** (INCI: Pentapeptide-3), **Syn-Ake** (INCI: Dipeptide Diaminobutyroyl Benzylamide Diacetate), **Inyline** (INCI: Acetyl Hexapeptide-25). These peptides block the ACh receptor, the activation of which leads to the entry of sodium ions inside the muscle cell, which are necessary for the polarization of the membrane and the initiation of the contraction process.

similarly to Argireline® — it is essentially an elongated version of Argireline® consisting of eight amino acids.

Other peptides that also interfere with neuromuscular transmission, but in a different way, have emerged. Pentapeptide Leuphasyl® (INCI: Pentapeptide-18) mimics the action of enkephalin — it reduces excitation in the neuron by inhibiting the flow of calcium ions across the membrane and reduces Ca^{2+}-dependent release of the mediator.

Several peptides work at the level of the postsynaptic membrane — Vialox® (INCI: Pentapeptide-3), Syn-Ake® (INCI: Dipeptide Diaminobutyroyl Benzylamide Diacetate), and Inyline® (INCI: Acetyl Hexapeptide-25). They block the ACh receptor, which opens when bound to a mediator (ACh), and his "window" inside the muscle cell facilitates the entry of the sodium ions necessary to polarize the membrane and start the contraction process. Even though the ways of ACh receptor blockade are different, the result is the same: closed receptor → no sodium flow → no polarization → no muscle contraction (relaxation).

In addition to synthetic peptides, natural components with myorelaxant action can be found in cosmetics. For example, hibiscus seed extract (*Hibiscuses culentus L.*) is sold under the commercial name Myoxinol® (INCI: Hydrolyzed Hibiscus Esculentus Extract (and) Dextrin). It is not known in detail how it blocks signal transmission from neuron to muscle, but it demonstrates a relaxing effect.

Remember that "Botox-like" ingredients are effective only in expression lines but are powerless against static wrinkles. Therefore, in modern cosmetic products, "Botox-like" substances are combined with remodeling peptides that improve the quality of the dermal matrix and biomechanical properties of the skin.

Unfortunately, the actual situation is far from *in vitro* conditions. *In vivo*, a peptide must overcome an almost impenetrable barrier — the *stratum corneum*, which is extremely difficult. Despite promising results in cell culture studies, cosmetic "Botox-like" ingredients are inferior to natural botulinum toxin in terms of clinical efficacy in human studies. However, while their myorelaxant effect can still be potentiated with long-term use, they are powerless against hyperhidrosis.

"Botox-like" cosmetic products belong to the first generation of topical myorelaxants. None of the known and authorized for cometic use "Botox-like" peptides have any commonalities with botulinum toxin in structure, origin, or mechanism of action. They are called "Botox-like" because they can cause, to a limited extent, muscle relaxation.

1.2. Topical botulinum toxin

In 2012, Dr. Alastair Carruthers said: "Pay attention to topical botulinum toxin preparations. I think they will revolutionize the neurotoxin market." His statement sounded sensational at the time, but the progenitor of aesthetic botulinum therapy was not discussing displacing injectable forms with topical agents but expanding this method's possibilities. He turned out to be correct. Only a few years later, such technology appeared on the market. Still, it must be noted that several unsuccessful starts preceded it.

The Transdermal Corp. (Birmingham, Michigan, USA) was one of the first to announce the topical BoNT. The company, founded in August 2008, was initially focused on transdermal drug delivery systems. Its Ionic Nano Particle Technology (INParT™) allows encapsulation of large molecules such as collagen, stabilized (cross-linked) hyaluronic acid and its sodium salt, small in size but highly irritating benzoyl peroxide (an antimicrobial component in acne treatment formulations), local anesthetic lidocaine, and others. INParT™ technology, based on the formation of mixed 1–10-nm micelles with incorporated drug molecules, proved to be suitable for "packaging" botulinum toxin, ensuring its stabilization in the emulsion, which is highly relevant. The point is that, unlike a solution for injection, an emulsion has aqueous and oil phases combined with an emulsifier. In such an environment, the 3D conformation of protein molecules is disturbed, and they lose their biological activity. Encapsulation in micelles prevents the denaturation of botulinum toxin in an unfriendly emulsion environment.

Cream with natural botulinum toxin type A encapsulated by INParT™ technology, named CosmeTox, was designed for expression lines and hyperhidrosis (Chajchir A. et al., 2008; Collins A., Nasir A., 2010). Unlike the solution, the cream can be stored at room temperature, and its activity during the shelf life is not reduced.

Despite a promising start, CosmeTox has quietly left the market, and given that the only information about this product available online is at least ten years old, we can only speculate about the reasons. Perhaps one of the factors is insufficient therapeutic efficacy due to the poor passage of encapsulated botulinum toxin through the *stratum corneum*, which makes using this product for medical indications pointless. Another reason is the impossibility of using natural botulinum toxin in cosmetics since it is a drug.

Revance Therapeutics (Newark, California, USA) took a different approach. In its product, RT001, botulinum toxin is modified using the TransMTS™ technology, which involves attaching a peptide transfer vector to the botulinum toxin complex. This drug failed Phase 3 clinical trials, and the project was terminated in 2016.

However, the research of South Korean scientists (Lee B.K., 2019), which led to the development of a modified botulinum toxin named BoLCA (**Bo**tulinum toxin **L**ight **C**hain type **A**), succeeded in solving all three problems:

1. Stabilize the active component
2. Ensure that it is transported through the *stratum corneum* and into the target cell
3. Obtain approval for use in cosmetics (INCI: Methionyl p-Clostridium Botulinum Polypeptide-1 Hexapeptide-40)

The critical point here is that not the entire botulinum toxin complex was taken, but only its active part, the light chain. However, even this light chain has difficulty passing through the *stratum corneum*, as it is still large and water-soluble. Let's assume it managed to do so, another problem would still arise: how to bind to the target cell? Recall that the heavy chain provides binding to the cell receptor, which has a special domain for this purpose (see Part I, chapter 1). The light chain alone cannot do this. The developers found a solution by attaching to the light chain a synthetic peptide with a structure that repeats the receptor-binding site of the heavy chain. This peptide serves as a transfer vector through the *stratum corneum* because, being poorly soluble in water, it improves the diffusion of the light chain through the lipid barrier of the *stratum corneum*. Besides, it ensures the binding of the light chain to its receptor on the cell membrane and its direct entry into the cell cytoplasm (**Fig. V-2**). Inside the cell, the light chain detaches from the peptide vector and begins to work as the light chain of botulinum toxin type A should do — it destroys the SNAP-25. Therefore, unlike "Botox-like" peptides, the mechanism of BoLCA action is like that of natural botulinum toxin.

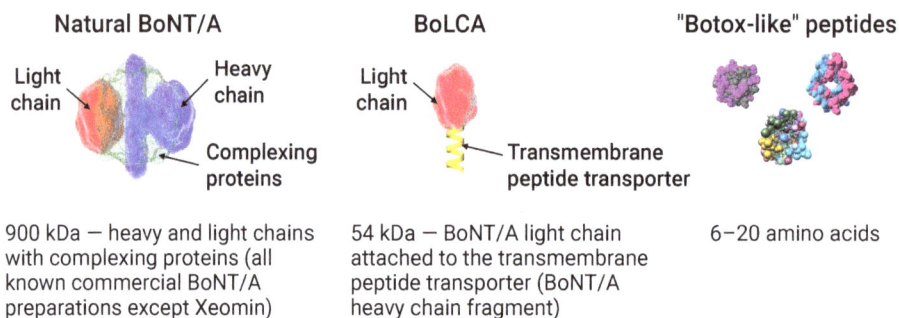

Natural BoNT/A	BoLCA	"Botox-like" peptides

Light chain — Heavy chain — Complexing proteins

Light chain — Transmembrane peptide transporter

900 kDa — heavy and light chains with complexing proteins (all known commercial BoNT/A preparations except Xeomin)

150 kDa — toxin heavy and light chains without complexing proteins (Xeomin)

54 kDa — BoNT/A light chain attached to the transmembrane peptide transporter (BoNT/A heavy chain fragment)

6–20 amino acids

	BoLCA	"BOTOX-LIKE" PEPTIDE
Structure	Modified BoNT light chain	Completely different from BoNT
Molecular mechanism of action and intracellular targets	The same as BoNT's	Different from BoNT
Effect	Disruption of signal (ACh) transmission from nerve endings to ACh-dependent cell	

Figure V-2. Comparison of BoLCA and "Botox-like" peptides with natural BoNT

BoLCA passes through the *stratum corneum* and ends up in the epidermis and dermis, interacting with various cells with BoNT receptors. Hence, there is a wide range of indications for its use (**Table V-1**).

As for the muscles, they are too deeply located to expect a pronounced myorelaxant effect from topical BoNT. In this respect, there is no alternative to injectable botulinum therapy, which delivers the neurotoxin to the right point in the right amount. But BoLCA works well in the superficial layers of the skin. Accordingly, the indications for topical botulinum toxin would be dermatologic problems, not increased muscle activity. An analogy can rather be drawn with multiple intradermal BoNT/A microinjections (see Part III), but the injection treatment belongs to the medical field, while the non-invasive topical application of BoLCA products belongs to the cosmetic field.

Table V-1. Clinical effects and indications for BoLCA use

TARGET	CLINICAL RESULT	INDICATIONS
Indirect action through the disruption of ACh and other mediators release (including pro-inflammatory mediators) in skin nerve endings		
Sweat gland cells	Reduced sweating	Excessive sweating
Sebocytes	Decreased sebosecretion	Seborrhea, seborrheic dermatitis, acne
Endothelial cells	Decreased NO production	Couperosis, rosacea, hematomas
Immune cells	Reduced release of pro-inflammatory mediators	Inflammation
Direct action on cells (established but poorly understood)		
Keratinocytes	Improved migration	Hyperkeratosis, erosions
Fibroblasts, myofibroblasts	Cell cycle regulation	Scars (prevention and treatment), full-thickness skin damage, age-related dermal atrophy

Résumé

"Botox-like" cosmetic products will perfectly complement injectable botulinum therapy and possibly prolong its clinical effect but will not replace it. They are all extremely weak myorelaxants and cannot be considered an alternative to BoNT injections. However, they have other beneficial properties related to their effect on epidermal and dermal cells.

The topical botulinum toxin BoLCA stands out in its wide range of clinical effects in the epidermis and dermis, which are characteristic of natural botulinum toxin. As for "Botox-like" peptides, their long-term use may help with wrinkle smoothing. However, this effect is likely due to other mechanisms of action and other cellular targets rather than the actual relaxation of mimic muscles.

Despite everything, "Botox-like" cosmetics have carved a niche in the cosmetic market, which is likely to remain and expand. The emergence of new "Botox-like" ingredients and ongoing research on modified forms of BoNT for topical application will ensure their rightful place in skincare (Saffarian P., Fooladi A.A.I., 2018).

References

Abdallah Hajj Hussein I., Dali Balta N., Jurjus R.A. et al. Rat model of burn wound healing: effect of Botox. J Biol Regul Homeost Agents 2012; 26(3): 389–400.

Ahn K.Y. Commentary: the effect of botulinum toxin type A injection on lower facial contouring evaluated using a three-dimensional laser scan. Dermatol Surg 2010; 36 Suppl 4: 2167.

Alam M., Barrett K.C., Hodapp R.M. et al. Botulinum toxin and the facial feedback hypothesis: can looking better make you feel happier? J Am Acad Dermatol 2008; 58(6): 1061–1072.

Almeida de A.T., Figueredo V., da Cunha A.L.G. et al. Consensus recommendations for the use of hyperdiluted calcium hydroxyapatite (Radiesse) as a face and body biostimulatory agent. Plast Reconstr Surg Glob Open 2019; 7(3): e2160.

Al-Qattan M.M., Al-Shanawani B.N., Alshomer F. Botulinum toxin type A: implications in wound healing, facial cutaneous scarring, and cleft lip repair. Ann Saudi Med 2013; 33(5): 482–488.

Anand C. Facial contouring with fillers, neuromodulators, and lipolysis to achieve a natural look in patients with facial fullness. J Drugs Dermatol 2016; 15(12): 1536–1542.

Artemenko A.R. Botulinum toxin type A in treating hyperhidrosis and other localized vegetative disorders. Injekzionnye Metody v Kosmetologii [Cosmetic Injections J] 2011; 1: 76.

Aydil B., Basaran B., Unsaler S., Suoglu Y. The use of botulinum toxin type A in masseteric muscle hypertrophy: long-term effects and lasting improvement. Kulak Burun Bogaz Ihtis Derg 2012; 22(5): 249–253.

Bae D.S., Koo D.H., Kim J.E. et al. Effect of botulinum toxin a on scar healing after thyroidectomy: a prospective double-blind randomized controlled trial. J Clin Med 2020; 9(3): 868.

Bagues A., Hu J., Alshanqiti I., Chung M.K. Neurobiological mechanisms of botulinum neurotoxin-induced analgesia for neuropathic pain. Pharmacol Ther 2024; 259: 108668.

Bansal C., Omlin K.J., Hayes C.M., Rohrer T.E. Novel cutaneous uses for botulinum toxin type A. J Cosmet Dermatol 2006; 5(3): 268–272.

Bartkowska P., Roszak J., Ostrowski H., Komisarek O. Botulinum toxin type A as a novel method of preventing cleft lip scar hypertrophy – a literature review. J Cosmet Dermatol 2020; 19(9): 2188–2193.

Becker W.J. Botulinum toxin in the treatment of headache. Toxins (Basel) 2020; 12(12): 803.

Beer K.R., Julius H., Dunn M., Wilson F. Remodeling of periorbital, temporal, glabellar, and crow's feet areas with hyaluronic acid and botulinum toxin. J Cosmet Dermatol 2014; 13(2): 143–150.

Bellows S., Jankovic J. Immunogenicity associated with botulinum toxin treatment. Toxins (Basel) 2019; 11(9): 491.

Berman B., Maderal A., Raphael B. Keloids and hypertrophic scars: pathophysiology, classification, and treatment. Dermatol Surg 2017; 43(Suppl 1): S3–S18.

Bharti J., Sonthalia S., Jakhar D. Mesotherapy with botulinum toxin for the treatment of refractory vascular and papulopustular rosacea. J Am Acad Dermatol 2018; 88(6): e295–e296.

Bi M., Sun P., Li D. et al. Intralesional injection of botulinum toxin type A compared with intralesional injection of corticosteroid for the treatment of hypertrophic scar and keloid: a systematic review and meta-analysis. Med Sci Monit 2019; 25: 2950–2958.

Binder W.J. Long-term effects of botulinum toxin type A (Botox) on facial lines: a comparison in identical twins. Arch Facial Plast Surg 2006; 8(6): 426–431.

Bloom B.S., Payongayong L., Mourin A., Goldberg D.J. Impact of intradermal abobotulinumtoxinA on facial erythema of rosacea. Dermatol Surg 2015; 41(1): 9–16.

Bosniak S., Cantisano-Zilkha M., Purewal B.K., Zdinak L.A. Combination therapies in oculofacial rejuvenation. Orbit 2006; 25(4): 319–326.

Boughdadi N.S., Sadek E.Y. Combination of botulinum toxin type A and fractional erbium-YAG laser in treatment of crow's feet. J Plast Reconstr Surg 2010; 34(2): 139–145.

Bowler P.J. Dermal and epidermal remodeling using botulinum toxin type A for facial, nonreducible, hyperkinetic lines: two case studies. J Cosmet Dermatol 2008; 7(3): 241–244.

Braccini F., Dohan Ehrenfest D.M. Advantages of combined therapies in cosmetic medicine for the treatment of face aging: botulinum toxin, fillers and mesotherapy. Rev Laringol Otol Rhinol 2010; 131(2): 1–8.

Brin M.F., Kirby R.S., Slavotinek A. et al. Pregnancy outcomes following exposure to onabotulinumtoxinA. Pharmacoepidem Drug Safety 2016; 25(2): 179–187.

Brin M.F., Nelson M., Ashourian N. et al. Update on non-interchangeability of botulinum neurotoxin products. Toxins (Basel) 2024; 16(6): 266.

Buddenkotte J., Steinhoff M. Recent advances in understanding and managing rosacea. F1000Res 2018; 2018 Dec 3:7:F1000 Faculty Rev-1885.

Callejas M.A., Grimalt R., Cladellas E. Hyperhydrosis update. Actas Dermosifiliogr 2010; 101(2): 110–118.

Calvisi L., Diaspro A., Sito G. Microbotox: a prospective evaluation of dermatological improvement in patients with mild-to-moderate acne and erythematotelangiectatic rosacea. J Cosmet Dermatol 2022; 21(9): 3747–3753.

Carloni R., Pechevy L., Postel F. et al. Is there a therapeutic effect of botulinum toxin on scalp alopecia? Physiopathology and reported cases: a systematic review of the literature. J Plast Reconstr Aesthet Surg 2020; 73(12): 2210–2216.

Carr W.W., Jain N., Sublett J.W. Immunogenicity of botulinum toxin formulations: potential therapeutic implications. Adv Ther 2021; 38(10): 5046–5064.

Carruthers A., Carruthers J., Dover J.S. et al. Procedures in Cosmetic Dermatology: Botulinum Toxin, 5th edition. Elsivier, 2022.

Carruthers A., Carruthers J., Monheit G.D. et al. Multicenter, randomized, parallel-group study of the safety and effectiveness of onabotulinumtoxinA and hyaluronic acid dermal fillers (24-mg/ml smooth, cohesive gel) alone and in combination for lower facial rejuvenation. Dermatol Surg 2010; 36(Suppl 4): 2121–2134.

Carruthers J., Burgess C., Day D. et al. Consensus recommendations for combined aesthetic interventions in the face using botulinum toxin, fillers, and energy-based devices. Dermatol Surg 2016; 42(5): 586–597.

Carruthers J., Carruthers A. A prospective, randomized, parallel-group study analyzing the effect of BTX-A (BOTOX) and nonanimal-sourced hyaluronic acid (NASHA, Restylane) in combination compared with NASHA (Restylane) alone in severe glabellar rhytides in adult female subjects: treatment of severe glabellar rhytides with a hyaluronic acid derivative compared with the derivative and BTX-A. Dermatol Surg 2003; 29(8): 802–809.

Carruthers J., Carruthers A. Botox use in the mid and lower face and neck. Semin Cutan Surg 2001; 20(2): 85–92.

Carruthers J., Carruthers A. Botulinum toxin and laser resurfacing for lines around the eyes. In: Management of Facial Lines and Wrinkles. Blitzer A., Binder W.J., Carruthers A. (eds.). Lippincott Williams & Wilkins, 2000, pp. 315–318.

Carruthers J., Carruthers A. Combining botulinum toxin injection and laser resurfacing for facial rhytides. In: Combined Therapy: BOTOX and CO2 Facial Laser Resurfacing. Coleman L.W. (ed.). Williams & Wilkins, 1998, pp. 235–243.

Carruthers J., Carruthers A. The effect of full-face broadband light treatments alone and in combination with bilateral crow's feet botulinum toxin type-A chemodenervation. Dermatol Surg 2004; 30(3): 355–366.

Carruthers J., Glogau R.G., Blitzer A. Facial Aesthetics Consensus Group Faculty. Advances in facial rejuvenation: botulinum toxin type A, hyaluronic acid dermal fillers, and combination therapies — consensus recommendations. Plast Reconstr Surg 2008; 121(5 Suppl): S5–S30.

Chajchir I., Modi P., Chajchir A. Novel topical BoNTA (CosmeTox, toxin type A) cream used to treat hyperfunctional wrinkles of the face, mouth, and neck. Aesthetic Plast Surg 2008; 32(5): 715–722; discussion 723.

Chang S.P., Tsai H.H., Chen W.Y. et al. The wrinkles soothing effect on the middle and lower face by intradermal injection of botulinum toxin type A. Int J Dermatol 2008; 47(12): 1287–1294.

Chen M., Yan T., Ma K. et al. Botulinum toxin type A inhibits α-smooth muscle actin and myosin II expression in fibroblasts derived from scar contracture. Ann Plast Surg 2016; 77(3): e46–e49.

Choi J.E., Werbel T., Wang Z. et al. Botulinum toxin blocks mast cells and prevents rosacea-like inflammation. J Dermatol Sci 2019; 93(1): 58–64.

Choudhury S., Baker M.R., Chatterjee S., Kumar H. Botulinum toxin: an update on pharmacology and newer products in development. Toxins (Basel) 2021; 13(1): 58.

Cohen-Letessier A. Controverse: la toxine botulique previentelle le vieillissement cutane? [Controversy: botulinum toxin, does it prevent cutaneous aging?] Ann Dermatol Venereol 2009; 136(Suppl 4): 89–91.

Coleman K.R., Carruthers J. Combination therapy with BOTOX and fillers: the new rejuvenation paradigm. Dermatol Ther 2006; 19(3): 177–188.

Collins A., Nasir A. Topical botulinum toxin. J Clin Aesthet Dermatol 2010; 3(3): 35–39.

Comella J.X., Molgo J., Faille L. Sprouting of mammalian motor nerve terminals induced by in vivo injection of botulinum type-D toxin and the functional recovery of paralysed neuromuscular junctions. Neurosci Lett 1993; 153(1): 61–64.

Cook B.E., Lucarelli M.J., Lemke B.N. Depressor supercilii muscle: anatomy, histology, and cosmetic implications. Ophthal Plast Reconstr Surg 2001; 17(6): 404–411.

Costa A.C.F., Silva E.C.D., Gondim D.V. Botulinum toxin in facial aesthetics affects the emotion process: a meta-analysis of randomized controlled trials. Clin Psychopharmacol Neurosci 2022; 20(4): 600–608.

Dailey R.A., Philip A., Tardie G. Long-term treatment of glabellar rhytides using onabotulinumtoxinA. Dermatol Surg 2011; 37(7): 918–928.

Dayan S.H., Ashourian N., Cho K. A pilot, double-blind, placebo-controlled study to assess the efficacy and safety of incobotulinumtoxinA injections in the treatment of rosacea. J Drugs Dermatol 2017; 16(6): 549–554.

Dayan S.H., Pritzker R.N., Arkins J.P. A new treatment regimen for rosacea: onabotulinumtoxinA. J Drugs Dermatol 2012; 11(12): 76–79.

Dayel S.B., Hussein R.S., Gafar H.H. The role of botulinum neurotoxin BoNT-A in the management of oily skin and acne vulgaris: a comprehensive review. Medicine (Baltimore) 2024; 103(8): e37208.

de Maio M. The minimal approach: an innovation in facial cosmetic procedures. Aesthetic Plast Surg 2004; 28(5): 295–300.

de Maio M. Basic and therapeutic aspects of botulinum and tetanus toxin. Presented at the Enhancing Aesthetics Conference, Italy, June 12–14, 2008.

de Maio M., Swift A., Signorini M., Fagien S. Aesthetic leaders in facial aesthetics consensus committee. Facial assessment and injection guide for botulinum toxin and injectable hyaluronic acid fillers: focus on the upper face. Plast Reconstr Surg 2017a; 140(2): e265–e276.

de Maio M., Wu W.T.L., Goodman G.J., Monheit G. Alliance for the future of aesthetics consensus committee. Facial assessment and injection guide for botulinum toxin and injectable hyaluronic acid fillers: focus on the lower face. Plast Reconstr Surg 2017b; 140(3): e393–e404.

Devlikamova F.I., Orlova O.R., Rakhimullina O.A., Rogozhin A.A. Multiple injections of BoNT/A: should we be afraid of consequences? Injekzionnye Metody v Kosmetologii [Cosmetic Injections JJ] 2011; 1: 22–26.

Diba V.C., Cormack G.C., Burrows N.P. Botulinum toxin is helpful in aquagenic palmoplantar keratoderma. Br J Dermatol 2005; 152(2): 394–395.

Dolly J., Aoki K. The structure and mode of action of different botulinum toxins. Eur J Neurol 2006; 13: 1–9.

Dover J.S., Monheit G., Greener M., Pickett A. Botulinum toxin in aesthetic medicine: myths and realities. Dermatol Surg 2018; 44(2): 249–260.

Durham P.L. CGRP receptor antagonists: a new choice for acute treatment of migraine? Curr Opin Investig Drugs 2004; 5(7): 731–735.

Durham P.L., Cady R. Regulation of calcitonin gene-related peptide secretion from trigeminal nerve cells by botulinum toxin type A: implications for migraine therapy. Headache 2004; 44: 35–42.

Eleowa S.A., Zidan S.M. Combination of botulinum toxin type A and hyaluronic acid filler for treatment of moderate to severe glabellar rhytides: results of one year follow up. Life Sci J 2013; 10(4): 1835–1840.

Engel E.R., Ham J.A. Amelioration of trichotillomania with onabotulinumtoxinA for chronic migraine. BMJ Case Rep 2023; 16(2): e254006.

English R.S., Ruiz S. Use of botulinum toxin for androgenic alopecia: a systematic review. Skin Appendage Disord 2022; 8(2): 93–100.

Erdil D., Manav V., Türk C.B. et al. The clinical effect of botulinum toxin on pigmentation. Int J Dermatol 2023; 62(2): 250–256.

Eviatar J., Lo C., Kirszrot J. Radiesse: advanced techniques and applications for a unique and versatile implant. Plast Reconstr Surg 2015; 136(5 Suppl): 164–170.

Fabi S.G., Goldman M.P., Mills D.C. et al. Combining microfocused ultrasound with botulinum toxin and temporary and semi-permanent dermal fillers: safety and current use. Dermatol Surg 2016; 42(Suppl 2): S168–S176.

Fiedler L.S., Burk F. Treatment of Frey syndrome with botulinum toxin-A: a practical approach from Minor's test to injection. J Maxillofac Oral Surg 2024; 23(2): 337–339.

Finzi E. Botulinum toxin treatment for depression: a new paradigm for psychiatry. Toxins (Basel) 2023; 15(5): 336.

Finzi E., Wasserman E. Treatment of depression with botulinum toxin A: a case series. Dermatol Surg 2006; 32(5): 645–650.

Flavio A. Botulinum Toxin for Facial Harmony. Quintessence Pub Co., 1st edition, 2018.

Freshwater M.F. Botulinum toxin for scars: can it work, does it work, is it worth it? J Plast Reconstr Aesthet Surg 2013; 66(3): 92–93.

Friedland S., Burde R.M. Porcelinizing discolorization of the periocular skin following botulinum A toxin injections. J Neuroophthalmol 1996; 16(1): 70–72.

Fujimura T., Hotta M. The preliminary study of the relationship between facial movements and wrinkle formation. Skin Res Technol 2012; 18(2): 219–224.

Gassner H.G., Brissett A.E., Otley C.C. et al. Botulinum toxin to improve facial wound healing: a prospective, blinded, placebo-controlled study. Mayo Clin Proc 2006; 81(8): 1023–1028.

Gauglitz G.G., Bureik D., Dombrowski Y. et al. Botulinum toxin A for the treatment of keloids. Skin Pharmacol Physiol 2012; 25(6): 313–318.

Gerasimov M.M. The basics of skull facial reconstruction. Soviet Science, 1949.

Glaser A., Naumann M. Botulinum neurotoxin in the management of hyperhidrosis and other hypersecretory disorders. In: Botulinum Toxin. Jankovic J., Albanese A., Zouhair Atassi M. et al. (eds.). W.B. Saunders, 2009, pp. 308–323.

Goldman A., Wollina U. Facial rejuvenation for middle-aged women: a combined approach with minimally invasive procedures. Clin Interv Aging 2010; 23(5): 293–299.

Goodman G.J. The use of botulinum toxin as primary or adjunctive treatment for postacne and traumatic scarring. J Cutan Aesthet Surg 2010; 3(2): 90–92.

Hamblin M. Mechanisms of low-level light therapy. Proceedings of SPIE — The International Society for Optical Engineering 2006; 6140: 1–12.

Han C., Park G.Y., Wang S.M. et al. Can botulinum toxin improve mood in depressed patients? Expert Rev Neurother 2012; 12(9): 1049–1051.

Hanna E., Pon K. Updates on botulinum neurotoxins in dermatology. Am J Clin Dermatol 2020; 21(2): 157–162.

Hartl D.M., Julieron M., LeRidant A.M. et al. Botulinum toxin A for quality of life improvement in post-parotidectomy gustatory sweating (Frey's syndrome). J Laryngol Otol 2008; 122(10): 1100–1104.

He G., Yang Q., Wu J. et al. Treating rosacea with botulism toxin: protocol for a systematic review and meta-analysis. J Cosmet Dermatol 2024; 23(1): 44–61.

Henning M.A.S., Bouazzi D., Jemec G.B.E. Treatment of hyperhidrosis: an update. Am J Clin Dermatol 2022; 23(5): 635–646.

Hornberger J., Grimes K., Naumann M. et al. Recognition, diagnosis, and treatment of primary focal hyperhidrosis. J Am Acad Dermatol 2004; 51(2): 274–286.

Hu L., Zou Y., Chang S.J. et al. Effects of botulinum toxin on improving facial surgical scars: a prospective, split-scar, double-blind, randomized controlled trial. Plast Reconstract Surg 2018; 141(3): 646–650.

Jabbari B. Basics of structure and mechanisms of function of botulinum toxin — how does it work? In: Botulinum toxin treatment. Springer, 2018, pp. 11–17.

Jung J.A., Kim B.J., Kim M.S. et al. Protective effect of botulinum toxin against ultraviolet-induced skin pigmentation. Plast Reconstr Surg 2019; 144(2): 347–356.

Kandhari R., Kaur I., Gupta J., Al-Niaimi F. Microdroplet botulinum toxin: a review. J Cutan Aesthet Surg 2022; 15(2): 101–107.

Kang S.M., Feneran A., Kim J.K. et al. Exaggeration of wrinkles after botulinum toxin injection for forehead horizontal lines. Ann Dermatol 2011; 23(2): 217–221.

Karamfilov T., Konrad H., Karte K., Wollina U. Lower relapse rate of botulinum toxin A therapy for axillary hyperhidrosis by dose increase. Arch Dermatol 2000; 136(4): 487–490.

Karpova E.I., Gubanova E.I. Volumetric correction of the suborbital area. Injekzionnye Metody v Kosmetologii [Cosmetic Injections J] 2010; 3: 16–21.

Karpova E.L. Photodynamic therapy in cosmetic anti-age programs. Apparatnaya Kosmetologiya [Hardware Cosmetology J] 2018; 1–2: 92–98.

Karu T. Mitochondrial mechanisms of photobiomodulation in context of new data about multiple roles of ATP. Photomed Laser Surg 2010; 28(2): 159–160.

Kasyanju Carrero L.M., Ma W.W., Liu H.F. et al. Botulinum toxin type A for the treatment and prevention of hypertrophic scars and keloids: updated review. J Cosmet Dermatol 2019; 18(1): 10–15.

Kattimani V., Tiwari R.V.C., Gufran K. et al. Botulinum toxin application in facial esthetics and recent treatment indications (2013–2018). J Int Soc Prev Community Dent 2019; 9(2): 99–105.

Katz B., Miledi E. A study of synaptic transmission in the absence of nerve impulses. J Physiol 1967; 192(2): 407–436.

Kim D., Park J.H., Favero V. et al. Effect of botulinum toxin injection on asymmetric lower face with chin deviation. Toxins (Basel) 2020; 12(7): 456.

Kim Y.S., Lee H.J., Cho S.H. et al. Early postoperative treatment of thyroidectomy scars using botulinum toxin: a split-scar, double-blind randomized controlled trial. Wound Repair Regen 2014; 22(5): 605–612.

Klein A.W., Fagien S. Hyaluronic acid fillers and botulinum toxin type A: rationale for their individual and combined use for injectable facial rejuvenation. Plast Reconstr Surg 2007; 120(6 Suppl): 81–88.

Ko C.P. Do nerve terminal sprouts contribute to functional recovery from botulinum neurotoxin A? J Physiol 2008; 586(13): 3021.

Koerte I.K., Schroeder A.S., Fietzek U.M. et al. Muscle atrophy beyond the clinical effect after a single dose of onabotulinumtoxinA injected in the procerus muscle: a study with magnetic resonance imaging. Dermatol Surg 2013; 39(5): 761–765.

Kruse D., Mackanos M., O'Connell-Rodwell C. et al. Short-duration-focused ultrasound stimulation of Hsp70 expression in vivo. Phys Med Biol 2008; 53(13): 3641–3660.

Kurzen H., Berger H., Jäger C. et al. Phenotypical and molecular profiling of the extraneuronal cholinergic system of the skin. J Invest Dermatol 2004; 123(5): 937–949.

Kwon K.H., Shin K.S., Yeon S.H., Kwon D.G. Application of botulinum toxin in maxillofacial field: part I. Bruxism and square jaw. Plast Reconstruct Surg 2019; 41(1): 38.

Laccourreye O., Muscatello L., Gutierrez-Fonseca R. et al. Severe Frey syndrome after parotidectomy: treatment with botulinum neurotoxin type A. Ann Otolaryngol Chir Cervicofac 1999; 116(3): 137–142.

Lakraj A.A.D., Moghimi N., Jabbari B. Hyperhidrosis: anatomy, pathophysiology and treatment with emphasis on the role of botulinum toxins. Toxins (Basel) 2013; 5(4): 821–840.

Landau M. Combination of chemical peelings with botulinum toxin injections and dermal fillers. J Cosmet Dermatol 2006; 5(2): 121–126.

Laskawi R., Drobik C., Schönebeck C. Up-to-date report of botulinum toxin type A treatment in patients with gustatory sweating (Frey's syndrome). Laryngoscope 1998; 108(3): 381–384.

Le Louarn C. Can the botulinum toxin prevent aging? Ann Dermatol Venereol 2009a; 136(Suppl 4): S92–S103.

Le Louarn C. Vieillissement musculaire et son implication dans le viellissement facial: le concept du Face Recurve. [Muscular aging and its involvement in facial aging: the Face Recurve concept.] Ann Dermatol Venereol 2009b; 136(Suppl 4): 67–72.

Le Louarn C. The deep cervical fascia neck lift. Ann Chir Plast Esthet 2024; 69(1): 101–108.

Le Louarn C., Buthiau D., Buis J. Structural aging: the facial recurve concept. Aesthetic Plast Surg 2007a; 31(3): 213–218.

Le Louarn C., Buthiau D., Buis J. The face recurve concept: medical and surgical applications. Aesthetic Plast Surg 2007b; 31(3): 219–231; discussion 232.

Lebeda F.J., Cer R.Z., Stephens R.M., Mudunuri U. Temporal characteristics of botulinum neurotoxin therapy. Expert Rev Neurother 2010; 10(1): 93–103.

Ledda C., Artusi C.A. Tribolo A. et al. Time to onset and duration of botulinum toxin efficacy in movement disorders. J Neurol 2022; 269(7): 3706–3712.

Lee B.K. BoLCA: second-generation cosmetic myorelaxants, or topical botulinum therapy for age-related skin changes. Cosmetics & Medicine 2019; 2: 32–38.

Lee B.K. Topical botulinum toxin for skin lightening: rationale and practical recommendations. Cosmetics & Medicine 2020; 1: 61.

Levy P.M. The "Nefertiti lift": a new technique for specific re-contouring of the jawline. J Cosmet Laser Ther 2007; 9(4): 249–252.

Li K., Meng F., Li Y.R. et al. Application of nonsurgical modalities in improving facial aging. Int J Dent 2022; 2022: 8332631.

Li Y., Liao M., Zhu Y. et al. Hyaluronic acid compound filling plus mesotherapy vs botulinum toxin A for the treatment of horizontal neck lines: a multicenter, randomized, evaluator-blinded, prospective study in Chinese subjects. Aesthet Surg J 2022; 42(4): NP230–NP241.

Li Y.H., Yang J., Zheng Z. et al. Botulinum toxin type A attenuates hypertrophic scar formation via the inhibition of TGF-beta1/Smad and ERK pathways. J Cosmet Dermatol 2021; 20(5): 1374–1380.

Li Z.J., Park S.B., Sohn K.C. et al. Regulation of lipid production by acetylcholine signalling in human sebaceous glands. J Dermatol Sci 2013; 72(2): 116–122.

Liang Y., Liu B., Li X., Wang P. Multivariate pattern classification of facial expressions based on large-scale functional connectivity. Front Hum Neurosci 2018; 12: 94.

Liu A., Moy R.L., Ozog D.M. Current methods employed in the prevention and minimization of surgical scars. Dermatol Surg 2011; 37(12): 1740–1746.

Maeshige N., Terashi H., Aoyama M. et al. Effect of ultrasound irradiation on alpha-SMA and TGF-beta1 expression in human fibroblasts. Kobe J Med Sci 2011; 56(6): E242–E252.

Martin M.U., Frevert J., Tay C.M. Complexing protein-free botulinum neurotoxin A formulations: implications of excipients for immunogenicity. Toxins (Basel) 2024; 16(2): 101.

Martires K.J., Fu P., Polster A.M. et al. Factors that affect skin aging: a cohort-based survey on twins. Arch Dermatol 2009; 145(12): 1375–1379.

McConaghy J.R., Fosselman D. Hyperhidrosis: management options. Am Fam Physician 2018; 97(11): 729–734.

Messikh R., Atallah L., Aubin F., Humbert P. Botulinum toxin in disabling dermatological diseases. Ann Dermatol Venereol 2009; 136(Suppl 4): S129–S136.

Meylan E., Tschopp J., Karin M. Intracellular pattern recognition receptors in the host response. Nature 2006; 442(7098): 39–44.

Mole B. Accordion wrinkle treatment through the targeted use of botulinum toxin injections. Aesthetic Plast Surg 2014; 38(2): 419–428

Mole B. Scratched faces: treatment of dynamic facial wrinkles through the simultaneous combined use of botulinum toxin A and hyaluronic acid. Ann Chir Plast Esthet 2012; 57(3): 194–201.

Moon H., Fundaro S.P., Goh C.L. et al. A review on the combined use of soft tissue filler, suspension threads, and botulinum toxin for facial rejuvenation. J Cutan Aesthet Surg 2021; 14(2): 147–155.

Nanda S., Bansal S. Upper face rejuvenation using botulinum toxin and hyaluronic acid fillers. Indian J Dermatol Venereol Leprol 2013; 79(1): 32–40.

Nassar A., Abdel-Aleem H., Samir M., Khattab F.M. Efficacy of botulinum toxin A injection in the treatment of androgenic alopecia: a comparative controlled study. J Cosmet Dermatol 2022; 21(10): 4261–4268.

Nawrocki S., Cha J. Botulinum toxin: pharmacology and injectable administration for the treatment of primary hyperhidrosis. J Am Acad Dermatol 2020; 82(4): 969–979.

Nestor M.S., Fischer D.L., Arnold D. "Masking" our emotions: botulinum toxin, facial expression, and well-being in the age of COVID-19. J Cosmet Dermatol 2020; 19(9): 2154–2160.

Nikolis A., Enright K.M., Rudolph C., Cotofana S. Temporal volume increase after reduction of masseteric hypertrophy utilizing incobotulinumtoxin type A. J Cosmet Dermatol 2020; 19(6): 1294–1300.

Odo M.E., Odo L.M., Farias R.V. et al. Botulinum toxin for the treatment of menopausal hot flushes: a pilot study. Dermatol Surg 2011; 37(11): 1579–1583.

Oh S.H., Lee Y., Seo Y.J. et al. The potential effect of botulinum toxin type A on human dermal fibroblasts: an in vitro study. Dermatol Surg 2012; 38(10): 1689–1694.

Okada H.C., Alleyne B., Varghai K. et al. Facial changes caused by smoking: a comparison between smoking and nonsmoking identical twins. Plast Reconstr Surg 2013;132(5): 1085–1092.

Okuda I. 3D CT images allow the depiction of the state of facial muscles and facial aging. Training course at Radiology Society of North America, 2010.

O'Neill J.P., Condron C., Curran A., Walsh A. Lucja Frey — historical relevance and syndrome review. Surgeon 2008; 6(3): 178–181.

Owsley J.Q., Roberts C.L. Some anatomical observations on midface aging and long-term results of surgical treatment. Plast Reconstr Surg 2008; 121(1): 258–268.

Padda I.S., Tadi P. Botulinum Toxin. StatPearls [Internet], 2023; StatPearls Publishing, 2024.

Park J.K., Hyun K., Moon M.H., Lee J. Surgical treatment of facial blushing: patient selection and operative technique (retrospective observational study). Medicine (Baltimore) 2022; 101(27): e29808.

Park K.Y., Kwon H.J., Kim J.M. et al. A pilot study to evaluate the efficacy and safety of treatment with botulinum toxin in patients with recalcitrant and persistent erythematotelangiectatic rosacea. Ann Dermatol 2018; 30(6): 688–693.

Parsagashvili E.Z. Combination of botulinum therapy and biorevitalization with IAL-System and IAL-System ACP. Injekzionnye Metody v Kosmetologii [Cosmetic Injections J] 2010; 2: 74–75.

Peck M.W., Smith T.J., Anniballi F. et al. Historical perspectives and guidelines for botulinum neurotoxin subtype nomenclature. Toxins (Basel) 2017; 9: 38.

Peskova I.V. Fillers and botulinum toxin — "star duet" of aesthetic medicine. Injekzionnye Metody v Kosmetologii [Cosmetic Injections J] 2014; 3: 57.

Quatela V.C., Ahmedli N.N. The selection of facelift approach on the basis of midfacial ptosis. Facial Plast Surg 2021; 37(2): 149–159.

Rainer B.M., Kang S., Chien A.L. Rosacea: epidemiology, pathogenesis, and treatment. Dermatoendocrinol 2017; 9(1): e1361574.

Rainer B.M., Thompson K.G., Antonescu C. et al. Characterization and analysis of the skin microbiota in rosacea: a case-control study. Am J Clin Dermatol 2020; 21(1): 139–147.

Rauso R., Lo Giudice G., Tartaro G. et al. Botulinum toxin type A injections for masticatory muscles hypertrophy: A systematic review. J Craniomaxillofac Surg 2022; 50(1): 7–18.

Rho N.K., Gil Y.C. Botulinum neurotoxin type A in the treatment of facial seborrhea and acne: evidence and a proposed mechanism. Toxins (Basel) 2021; 13(11): 817.

Rivkin A., Binder W.J. Long-term effects of onabotulinumtoxinA on facial lines: a 19-year experience of identical twins. Dermatol Surg 2015; 41(Suppl 1): S64–S66.

Robinson A.J., Khadim M.F., Khan K. Keloid scars and treatment with botulinum toxin type A: the Belfast experience. J Plast Reconstr Aesthet Surg 2013; 66(3): 439–440.

Rogozhin A.A., Pang K.K., Bukharaeva E. et al. Recovery of mouse neuromuscular junctions from single and repeated injections of botulinum neurotoxin A. J Physiol 2008; 586(13): 3163–3182.

Rose A.E., Goldberg D.J. Safety and efficacy of intradermal injection of botulinum toxin for the treatment of oily skin. Dermatol Surg 2013; 39(3 Pt 1): 443–448.

Rzany B., Dill-Muller D., Grablowitz D. et al. Repeated botulinum toxin A injections for the treatment of lines in the upper face: a retrospective study of 4,103 treatments in 945 patients. Dermatol Surg 2007; 33(1): 18–25.

Saffarian P., Fooladi A.A.I. Topical botulinum toxin: a non-invasive way for treatment of muscle disorders. Curr Drug Deliv 2018; 15(10): 1375–1380.

Salame N., Eber A.E., Dover J. DaxibotulinumtoxinA-lanm (Daxxify™): a comprehensive overview. Skin Therapy Lett 2023; 28(4): 1–3.

Scala J., Vojvodic A., Vojvodic P. et al. Botulin toxin use in rosacea and facial flushing treatment. Open Access Maced J Med Sci 2019; 7(18): 2985–2987.

Scott A.B., Honeychurch D., Brin M.F. Early development history of Botox (onabotulinumtoxinA). Medicine (Baltimore) 2023; 102(S1): e32371.

Shah A.R. Use of intradermal botulinum toxin to reduce sebum production and facial pore size. J Drugs Dermatol 2008; 7(9): 847–850.

Sharova A.A., Saromytskaya A.N. Paradoxes of aesthetic botulinum therapy. Injekzionnye Metody v Kosmetologii [Cosmetic Injections J] 2014; 1: 44.

Sherris D.A., Gassner H.G. Botulinum toxin to minimize facial scarring. Facial Plast Surg 2002; 18(1): 35–39.

Shim W.H., Yoon S.H., Park J.H. et al. Effect of botulinum toxin type A injection on lower facial contouring evaluated using a three-dimensional laser scan. Dermatol Surg 2010; 36(Suppl 4): 2161–2166.

Shon U., Kim M.H., Lee D.Y. et al. The effect of intradermal botulinum toxin on androgenetic alopecia and its possible mechanism. J Am Acad Dermatol 2020; 83(6): 1838–1839.

Shuo L., Ting Y., KeLun W. et al. Efficacy and possible mechanisms of botulinum toxin treatment of oily skin. J Cosmet Dermatol 2019; 18(2): 451–457.

Singh S., Neema S., Vasudevan B. A pilot study to evaluate effectiveness of botulinum toxin in treatment of androgenetic alopecia in males. J Cutan Aesthet Surg 2017; 10(3): 163–167.

Small R. Botulinum toxin injection for facial wrinkles. Am Fam Physician 2014; 90(3): 168–175.

Sohrabi C., Goutos I. The use of botulinum toxin in keloid scar management: a literature review. Scars Burn Heal 2020; 6: 2059513120926628.

Song W.C., Hu K.S., Kim H.J. et al. A study of the secretion mechanism of the sebaceous gland using three-dimensional reconstruction to examine the morphological relationship between the sebaceous gland and the arrector pili muscle in the follicular unit. Br J Dermatol 2007; 157(2): 325–330.

Srinoulprasert Y., Wanitphakdeedecha R. Antibody-induced botulinum toxin treatment failure: a review and novel management approach. J Cosmet Dermatol 2020; 19(10): 2491–2496.

Steinhoff M., Schmelz M., Schauber J. Facial erythema of rosacea — aetiology, different pathophysiologies and treatment options. Acta Derm Venereol 2016; 96(5): 579–586.

Sulk M., Seeliger S., Aubert J. et al. Distribution and expression of non-neuronal transient receptor potential (TRPV) ion channels in rosacea. J Invest Dermatol 2012; 132(4): 1253–1262.

Sundaram H., Liew S., Signorini M. et al. Global Aesthetics Consensus Group. Global aesthetics consensus: hyaluronic acid fillers and botulinum toxin type A — recommendations for combined treatment and optimizing outcomes in diverse patient populations. Plast Reconstr Surg 2016a; 137(5): 1410–1423.

Sundaram H., Signorini M., Liew S. et al. Global Aesthetics Consensus Group: botulinum toxin type A — evidence-based review, emerging concepts, and consensus recommendations for aesthetic use, including updates on complications. Plast Reconstr Surg 2016b; 137(3): e518–e529.

Surovovykh S.V., Orlova O.R., Saxonova E.V. Facial asymmetry. Minimally invasive correction of the consequences of facial nerve lesions. Injekzionnye Metody v Kosmetologii [Cosmetic Injections J] 2012; 3: 31–40.

Takahashi K.H., Utiyama T.O., Bagatin E. et al. Efficacy and safety of botulinum toxin for rosacea with positive impact on quality of life and self-esteem. Int J Dermatol 2024; 63(5): 590–596.

Tollefson T.T., Senders C.M., Sykes J.M., Byorth P.J. Botulinum toxin to improve results in cleft lip repair. Arch Facial Plast Surg 2006; 8(3): 221–222.

Tomkins S.S. The role of facial response in the experience of emotion: a reply to Tourangeau and Ellsworth. J Personal Soc Psychol 1981; 40: 355–357.

Ulashchik V.S., Timoshenko O.N. Influence of physical factors on morphofunctional state of cell culture. Voprosy Kurortologii, Physiotherapii i Lechebnoy Physcultury [Issues of Resortology, Physiotherapy and Therapeutic Physical Training] 2008; 3: 48–51.

Uyesugi B., Lippincott B., Dave S. Treatment of a painful keloid with botulinum toxin type A. Am J Phys Med Rehabil 2010; 89(2): 153–155.

Viera M.H., Amini S., Valins W., Berman B. Innovative therapies in the treatment of keloids and hypertrophic scars. J Clin Aesthet Dermatol 2010; 3(5): 20–26.

Vladimirov Y.A., Osipov A.N., Klebanov G.I. Photobiological principles of therapeutic applications of laser radiation. Biochemistry (Mosc) 2004; 69(1): 81–90.

Vlahovic T.C. Plantar hyperhidrosis: an overview. Clin Podiatr Med Surg 2016; 33(3): 441–451.

Vorkamp T., Foo F.J., Khan S. et al. Hyperhidrosis: evolving concepts and a comprehensive review. Surgeon 2010; 8(5): 287–292.

Walker T.J., Dayan S.H. Comparison and overview of currently available neurotoxins. J Clin Aesthet Dermatol 2014; 7(2): 31–39.

Wang F., Garza L.A., Kang S. et al. In vivo stimulation of de novo collagen production caused by cross-linked hyaluronic acid dermal filler injections in photodamaged human skin. Arch Dermatol 2007; 143(2): 155–163.

Welch M.J., Purkiss J.R., Foster K.A. Sensitivity of embryonic rat dorsal root ganglia neurons to Clostridium botulinum neurotoxins. Toxicon 2000; 38(2): 245–258.

West T.B., Alster T.A. Effect of botulinum toxin type A on movement-associated rhytides following CO2 laser resurfacing. Dermatol Surg 1999; 25(4): 259–261.

Wilson A.M. Use of botulinum toxin type A to prevent widening of facial scars. Plast Reconstr Surg 2006; 117(6): 1758–1766.

Wollina U., Payne C.R. Aging well the role of minimally invasive aesthetic dermatological procedures in women over 65. J Cosmet Dermatol 2010; 9(1): 50–58.

Wollmer M.A., de Boer C., Kalak N. et al. Facing depression with botulinum toxin: a randomized controlled trial. J Psychiatr Res 2012, 46(5): 574–581.

Woo Y.R., Lim J.H., Cho D.H., Park H.J. Rosacea: molecular mechanisms and management of a chronic cutaneous inflammatory condition. Int J Mol Sci 2016; 17(9): 1562.

Wright E., Fetsko L. Botulinum toxin type A injections for pediatric spasticity: keeping our patients informed and practices safe. J Pediatr Rehabil Med 2021;14(2):199–211.

Xiao Z., Qu G. Effects of botulinum toxin type A on collagen deposition in hypertrophic scars. Molecules 2012; 17(2): 2169–2177.

Xiao Z., Zhang F., Cui Z. Treatment of hypertrophic scars with intralesional botulinum toxin type A injections: a preliminary report. Aesthet Plast Surg 2009; 33(3): 409–412.

Xiaoxue W., Xi C., Zhibo X. Effects of botulinum toxin type A on expression of genes in keloid fibroblasts. Aesthet Surg J 2014; 34(1): 154–159.

Yamasaki K., Di Nardo A., Bardan A. et al. Increased serine protease activity and cathelicidin promotes skin inflammation in rosacea. Nat Med 2007; 13(8): 975–980.

Yamauchi P.S., Lask G., Lowe N.J. Botulinum toxin type A gives adjunctive benefit to periorbital laser resurfacing. J Cosmet Laser Ther 2004; 6(3): 145–148.

Yao B., Chen W., Wu S. et al. Er:YAG laser combined with botulinum toxin A for patients with local syringomas: a preliminary report. J Cosmet Dermatol 2023; 22(10): 2721–2728.

Yi K.H., Lee J.H., Hu H.W., Kim H.J. Anatomical proposal for botulinum neurotoxin injection for glabellar frown lines. Toxins (Basel) 2022; 14(4): 268.

Yi K.H., Lee J.H., Seo K.K., Kim H.J. anatomical proposal for botulinum neurotoxin injection for horizontal forehead lines. Plast Reconstr Surg 2024; 153(2): e322–e325.

Yiannakopoulou E. Serious and long-term adverse events associated with the therapeutic and cosmetic use of botulinum toxin. Pharmacology 2015; 95(1–2): 65–69.

Yue S., Ju M., Su Z. A systematic review and meta-analysis: botulinum toxin A effect on postoperative facial scar prevention. Aesthetic Plast Surg 2022; 46(1): 395–405.

Yutskovskaya Y.A., Kizei I.N., Timoshenko E.V., Orlova O.R. Pathogenetic substantiation of the combination of botulinotherapy and hardware methods in cosmetology. Injekzionnye Metody v Kosmetologii [Cosmetic Injections J] 2011; 4: 44.

Yutskovskaya Y.A., Remenyuk M.G., Naumchik G.A. Clinical experience of botulinum toxin type A application in the therapy of rosacea. Cosmetics & Medicine 2016; 1: 72–75.

Zhang H., Tang K., Wang Y. et al. Use of botulinum toxin in treating rosacea: a systematic review. Clin Cosmet Investig Dermatol 2021; 14: 407–417.

Zhao P., Jin M., He N. et al. Clinical observation of ultrapulse CO_2 dot array laser combined with botulinum toxin type A injection in the treatment of hypertrophic scar. Panminerva Med 2020 Jul 27.

Zhibo X., Miaobo Z. Botulinum toxin type A affects cell cycle distribution of fibroblasts derived from hypertrophic scar. J Plast Reconstr Aesthet Surg 2008; 61(9): 1128–1129.

Zhibo X., Miaobo Z. Intralesional botulinum toxin type A injection as a new treatment measure for keloids. Plast Reconstr Surg 2009; 124(5): 275–277.

Zhou Y., Yu S., Zhao J. et al. Effectiveness and safety of botulinum toxin type A in the treatment of androgenetic alopecia. Biomed Res Int 2020; 2020: 1501893.

Ziade M., Domergue S., Batifol D. et al. Use of botulinum toxin type A to improve treatment of facial wounds: a prospective randomised study. J Plast Reconstr Aesthet Surg 2013; 66(2): 209–214.

Zimbler M., Undavia S. Update on the effect of botulinum toxin pretreatment on laser resurfacing results. Arch Facial Plast Surg 2012; 14(3): 156–158.

Zouboulis C.C., Baron J.M., Bohm M. et al. Frontiers in sebaceous gland biology and pathology. Exp Dermatol 2008; 17(6): 542–551.

www.ingramcontent.com/pod-product-compliance
Lightning Source LLC
Chambersburg PA
CBHW052020030426

42335CB00026B/3217